INTRODUCTION TO NURSING FOR FIRST YEAR STUDENTS

Sara Miller McCune founded SAGE Publishing in 1965 to support the dissemination of usable knowledge and educate a global community. SAGE publishes more than 1000 journals and over 800 new books each year, spanning a wide range of subject areas. Our growing selection of library products includes archives, data, case studies and video. SAGE remains majority owned by our founder and after her lifetime will become owned by a charitable trust that secures the company's continued independence.

Los Angeles | London | New Delhi | Singapore | Washington DC | Melbourne

INTRODUCTION TO NURSING
FOR
FIRST YEAR STUDENTS

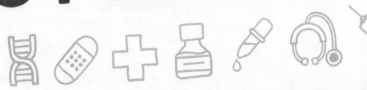

CALVIN MOORLEY

SAGE | LearningMatters

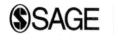

Learning Matters
An imprint of SAGE Publications Ltd
1 Oliver's Yard
55 City Road
London EC1Y 1SP

SAGE Publications Inc.
2455 Teller Road
Thousand Oaks, California 91320

SAGE Publications India Pvt Ltd
B 1/I 1 Mohan Cooperative Industrial Area
Mathura Road
New Delhi 110 044

SAGE Publications Asia-Pacific Pte Ltd
3 Church Street
#10-04 Samsung Hub
Singapore 049483

First published in 2020

Editor: Alex Clabburn
Development editor: Eleanor Rivers
Senior project editor: Chris Marke
Marketing manager: George Kimble
Cover design: Wendy Scott
Typeset by: C&M Digitals (P) Ltd, Chennai, India
Printed in the UK

Library of Congress Control Number: 2019947869

British Library Cataloguing in Publication Data

A catalogue record for this book is available from the British Library

ISBN 978-1-5264-3004-5
ISBN 978-1-5264-3005-2 (pbk)

At SAGE we take sustainability seriously. Most of our products are printed in the UK using responsibly sourced papers and boards. When we print overseas we ensure sustainable papers are used as measured by the PREPS grading system. We undertake an annual audit to monitor our sustainability.

Contents

About the editor and contributors

The editor

Calvin Moorley is an Associate Professor in Nursing Research and Diversity in Care in Adult Nursing in the School of Health and Social Care at London South Bank University. Dr Moorley was awarded the Mary Seacole Prize for Leadership in Nursing 2013/14 by Health Education England, recognising his work with ethnic minority groups. With a background in public health and diversity in care, his research focuses on the interplay of gender, culture, ethnicity and health. His most recent research includes knowledge, attitude and beliefs on sex among Black Africans; psychosexual experiences of FGM survivors and experience of stroke among Caribbean populations in the UK. He was the Guest Editor for the *Journal of Clinical Nursing* on LGBTI Health in 2017 and is an Associate Editor for the *Journal of Transcultural Nursing*. He has a keen interest in how health is theorised using social media platforms.

The contributors

Adebisi Adelaja, MA, PGCE and CELTA (Certificate in Teaching English to Speakers of Other Languages) qualified is a Learning Developer in the Centre for Research Informed Teaching (CRIT) at London South Bank University. Her 15 years' experience of teaching in further and higher education has involved facilitating students from a variety of subject disciplines to become independent learners. Her experience in academic practices includes working with nursing students from Foundation to Master's level to assist their application of theoretical and practical knowledge. Adebisi's current research interests include computerised forms of learning support, critical thinking and writing. She is a Fellow of the HEA (FHEA), a member of the Association for Learning Technology (ALT), and the Institute of Leadership and Management (ILM).

Stephen A Bowman, MA in Information Management and MSc in E-Learning, is the Learning and Teaching Librarian at London South Bank University. He is a Fellow of CILIP (FCLIP) and a Senior Fellow of the Higher Education Academy (SFHEA). He was an Associate Lecturer delivering education on 'Developing Digital Literacy', 'E-copyright' and 'The use of E-Resources', 'The Pedagogy of E-learning'. He has had articles published in the professional press and is a frequent reviewer for the *Information & Management* and *Library and Information Research* journals. He is a member of the International Committee of the 'European Conference on E-learning' (ECEL) and has an interest in student attitudes to learning resources following the introduction of student fees. His interests include the history of the book, film and cinema, and Prog Rock.

Marian Brown is currently an Academic Engagement Librarian at the University of Roehampton. Previously, she was an Information Skills Librarian at London South Bank University (LSBU), supporting the School of Health and Social Care across the two campuses in Southwark and Havering. While at LSBU, she achieved the Fellowship of the Higher Education Academy and was highly commended for Outstanding Student Support in the LSBU Staff Awards in 2018. She is passionate about finding innovative ways to support students and academics with information literacy, through the use of social media and learning technologies.

Xabi Cathala is a lecturer for the Institute of Vocational Learning in the School of Health and Social Care at London South Bank University. He is a registered nurse, specialised in Intensive Care Nursing. Passionate about research methods and information technology, he published a series of articles on how to appraise research and is undertaking a study on student nurses' use of social media. He has also been commissioned to write a series of articles to support newly qualified nurses. Xabi has an interest in equality and fairness in the health of minority individuals and groups. He speaks French and English.

Alexandra Costa is a senior staff nurse in an Intensive Care Unit in the private sector with more than 15 years' experience as a registered nurse. Having completed her nursing degree and worked in Portugal for more than eight years, she migrated to the UK and specialised in both High Dependency and Intensive Care Nursing (HDU/ITU) at City University, London. Alexandra is an infection control link nurse and supervises pre- and post-registration nurses in clinical practice. She has presented and participated at international conferences. She speaks Portuguese and English.

Nova Corcoran is a Senior Lecturer in Public Health and the course leader for the MSc in Public Health in the School of Care Sciences at the University of South Wales. She is a health promoter by background and the author of two health communication textbooks. Her research is centred on health communication and health promotion with minority groups, predominately using participatory and interactive research methods.

Jane Crussell is a Senior Lecturer and BSc Adult Nursing course director at London South Bank University. She is a registered nurse with a background in neurosurgery, maxillofacial surgery and chronic facial pain management. She has a research and teaching interest in end-of-life care in practice and education, and is Link Lecturer and Academic Lead at a local hospice. Her research interest is in student engagement within end-of-life care.

Marie Culloty is an Associate Professor for Adult Nursing and is lead for Adult Continuous Professional Development nursing in the School of Health and Social Care at London South Bank University. She is a registered nurse specialising in perioperative and anaesthetics nursing, and has over twenty years' experience in education of pre- and post-registration nurses. Marie's research interests focus on patient safety in acute settings.

Nicholas Gladstone is a Senior Lecturer in Adult Nursing in the School of Health and Social Care at London South Bank University. He is a registered nurse specialising in Trauma and Orthopaedic Nursing, and teaches postgraduate orthopaedic pathophysiology, fracture management and post-operative care following joint arthroplasty surgery. Nicholas has a keen interest in person-centred care, interprofessional practice and shared decision-making, and delivers education in this area on the pre-registration nursing programme. He publishes on clinical decision-making and nursing theory in various academic journals.

Debra Jones is a Senior Lecturer in Adult Nursing in the School of Health and Social Care at London South Bank University. She is a registered nurse who specialises in cardiothoracic nursing. Debra is the Course Director for the adult pre-registration nursing programme. Her lecturing portfolio includes pharmacology and medicines management.

Peter Jones is a Senior Lecturer at London South Bank University. He has an interest in care of the older adult and dementia. He is currently responsible for admissions to the pre-registration nursing programme. Peter qualified as a nurse in 1986 and has worked mainly in older adult care settings. Not only is he interested in the future of nursing, but also in its history.

Beverly Joshua is an experienced intensive care nurse, educator and researcher with a particular interest in professional nursing practice and improving students' learning ability through innovative educational strategy. She is the former Course Director for pre-registration adult nursing at London South Bank University. Her passion is to ensure that nursing students have the knowledge, skills, professionalism and clinical decision-making ability to deliver effective care to their patients. Dr Joshua's research investigated the correlation between students' learning approaches and their clinical decision-making while intervening to encourage the adoption of a deep approach to learning. She presented this study at the International Nursing Conference in Singapore (2015) and the European Doctoral Conference in Switzerland in 2016.

Sonia Kirby is a Senior Lecturer in Adult Nursing and Midwifery Department in the School of Health and Social Care at London South Bank University. She is a district nurse with a BSc (Hons) in Public Health and completed her MA in higher education. She is a senior fellow of the Higher Education Academy. Sonia leads on the Skills and Simulation courses in adult nursing, and is the lead for Public Health and Primary Care nursing education in the department.

Robert Murphy is a registered nurse and a Fellow of the Higher Education Academy. He was previously Senior Lecturer in Adult Nursing in the School of Health and Social Care at London South Bank University. Robert's academic interest and clinical practice focuses on end-of-life and hospice care.

Chioma Onyedinma-Ndubueze is a Senior Lecturer in Adult Nursing in the School of Health and Social Care at London South Bank University and a Fellow of the Higher

Education Academy. She is a registered nurse with many years' experience in medical and surgical nursing, and theories and practice of adult nursing. Chioma's teaching portfolio includes planning, developing and delivering education in individualised and person-centred care. Her specialist clinical practice is in the care of patients and families with haemoglobinopathies. Having developed standards and protocols for acute and community services for nurses, midwives and health visitors, she is a clinical nurse specialist in haemoglobinopathies. She has published articles on counselling patients and families with haemoglobinopathies. Chioma has developed health promotion resources on sickle cell disease. She has a special interest in widening participation in higher education and dyslexia, and supporting students with dyslexia in clinical practice.

Alwin Puthenpurakal is a Programme Lead and Senior Nurse Lecturer at BPP University. Having graduated from the University of Manchester and Queen Mary University of London, he has accumulated clinical experience in the field of intensive care nursing across London and Cambridge. Alwin has an interest in education management and healthcare leadership with the use of digital technology and has published in his clinical fields.

Mynesha Sankar is the Course Director for the Post Graduate Diploma in Adult Nursing Course in the School of Health and Social Care at London South Bank University. She is a registered nurse whose background is in Acute Respiratory Care. Her lecturing portfolio includes Mentorship and Care of the Deteriorating Patient. Mynesha is passionate about nurse education and has a research interest in the Theory Practice Gap in student nurses' education.

Pamela Thomas, MA (TESOL), has over 15 years' teaching experience in EFL (English as a Foreign Language), ESOL (English for Speakers of Other Languages) and EAP (English for Academic Purposes). She is a Learning Developer in the Centre for Research Informed Teaching (CRIT) at London South Bank University. She is a Fellow of the Higher Education Academy (FHEA), steering group committee member of the Association of Learning Developers in Higher Education (ALDinHE) and Certified Leading Practitioner of Learning Development. Pamela's research interest is in the field of academic literacy development, investigating how student writers in higher education transition with vocational qualifications and negotiate their way through the academic writing process within their subject-specific discipline.

Rosetta West, RN, EdD, is a Senior Lecturer at London South Bank University Adult Nursing and Midwifery Department in the School of Health and Social Care. Rosetta started her professional nursing journey in 1979 and has 40 years' practice and education experience in a variety of adult nursing settings. Pedagogical and clinical interests include gerontological nursing, pharmacology, diabetes management, the generalist perspective and education for sustainable development (ESD). Rosetta was awarded a professional doctorate for a thesis entitled 'Senior Nursing Lecturers' Understanding of Education for Sustainable Development: A Phenomenographic Study'. She investigated the understanding of her peers with the intention of translating this understanding into the nurse education curriculum and teaching framework.

Acknowledgements

I am in gratitude to all those who have mentored me in my career as a nurse clinically and academically. To all my co-authors, I have truly enjoyed working with you; thank you for making our writing and publication group a reality and success. I could not have completed writing this book without the support of Nick. Thank you for everything you do for me, understanding 'Calvin's world' and for keeping me grounded.

Introduction

Calvin Moorley

About this book: who is this book for?

This book is a result of the collective efforts of a group of nurses. The vision was to produce a text for first-year student nurses written by registered nurses that would help them to succeed in their nurse education. The book takes a practical approach to understanding nursing and caring for patients and different groups in society. One of the main reasons for this book is that most students encounter difficulties navigating the pre-registration nursing programme in the first year. Difficulties such as managing academic work/study and clinical practice, as well as having a family life, can be overwhelming. Our book aims to help students understand the level of academic and clinical work needed to be successful in the first year of their nursing programme. It is aimed at pre-registration nursing students and can be used by those in the first year of the Nursing Associate or Nursing Apprenticeship programme. Most of the scenarios used in this book are based on our real-world experience of working with patients and supporting nursing students. As a student nurse, you will make a contribution to the promotion of health, health protection and prevention of ill health, and this book helps you to perform in these areas. The book is mainly aimed at students undertaking the adult field. However, many of the chapters are applicable to those in mental health and learning disability. We hope that all who use this book will find it helpful, supportive and easy to understand, and that it complements their Year 1 learning and development.

Why *Introduction to Nursing for First Year Students*?

When I was a first-year nursing student I was told (by a mentor) that *I would never be a nurse.* On reflection, this was not because I did not like the profession or was not interested in learning. It was because I did not have the necessary skills, nor did I fully understand the extent of what it meant to care for someone or a group of people, particularly as a first-year nursing student. The reality of caring for someone who is vulnerable was difficult for me. Offering personal and intimate care was something I met with awkward expressions and mumbled words. I simply did not know how to navigate the nursing landscape. This book is aimed at helping first-year nursing students to develop skills and an understanding of what it is to be a nurse and to care using an evidence-based approach.

Choosing the title of this book was not very difficult as my vision was to support student nurses in their first year of study. Another reason for this stems from my years of experience (as a nurse and nurse educator) observing and hearing of the difficulties that first-year students encounter, and the fact that much of the attrition (the term used for students who withdraw or 'drop-out' from their course) in nursing occurs in the first year.

Nursing is the profession I hold close to my heart and the current workforce in the United Kingdom (UK) and globally is at critical levels, bordering on shortage. Therefore, this book is part of my contribution to keeping and sustaining our profession and ensuring that those who enter it have a solid foundation. The co-authors of this book, who are my colleagues in academic and clinical practice, share my passion and vision, one of which is for a professional and diverse nursing workforce. We have campaigned for a graduate workforce in the UK and are pleased that we can use our experience to develop this book to nurture future nurses. I am particularly proud that two of the authors in this book were educated outside the UK (France and Portugal), which demonstrates the important contribution of the global nursing workforce.

Book structure

The book is made up of ten chapters which are based on a logical order of the Year 1 nursing curriculum used at London South Bank University and in line with all current Nursing and Midwifery Council's standards for pre-registration nursing education.

Chapter 1 Professional values and practice This chapter is appropriate for adult, learning disability and mental health student nurses, and focuses on the various nursing settings – e.g. primary care, acute care and secondary care. It introduces the reader to the different models and frameworks utilised in nursing to deliver care. The chapter introduces the student to the use of reflection, and how personal and professional values are important in providing care to a diverse population. The focus is on developing an appreciation of the professional codes, ethical values and legal frameworks that underpin healthcare practice. Emphasis is upon knowledge, including ethical, legal and professional obligations to assess, plan, deliver and evaluate care, communicate findings, influence change and promote health, welfare and best practice.

Chapter 2 Introduction to research, resources and academic practices This chapter is designed to support students' academic practices for success in both adult, learning disability and mental health nursing. It introduces students to research, and finding academic resources and using the library. The chapter then moves to academic writing skills, covering areas such as brain-storming, essay planning, introducing critical thinking and analysis for writing.

Chapter 3 Communication in nursing This chapter is divided into two parts. The first part examines communication skills in nursing and working with diverse groups. It focuses on how adult and mental health and learning disability student nurses can develop their communication skills through health promotion – e.g. designing patient information literature. The second part looks at online communication: how to communicate electronically and use social media for professional purposes.

Chapter 4 Professional skills for adult nursing: Part 1 Assessment tools for clinical practice. This chapter aims to equip students with the essential and professional skills and knowledge that underpin contemporary nursing practice across the adult life span. The content is applicable to both adult and mental health and learning disability nursing students. It introduces key issues to provide safe and high-quality care, including the assessment of pressure areas, nutrition, risk of falling, continence, track and trigger systems and key basic interventions to manage these conditions. Students will be enabled to develop and expand their knowledge, practical ability and professional attitudes in promoting high-quality care through learning activities. It will encourage students to reflect on their own values and beliefs, and how this may affect their interactions with patients, carers and families.

Chapter 5 Professional skills for adult nursing: Part 2 Developing practical clinical skills. This chapter builds upon the student's previous learning (from Chapter 4) and enables them to develop and expand their understanding of nursing, as well their practice skills and knowledge. In addition, this chapter will provide theoretical knowledge which, when applied in practical settings, will improve and enhance care to patients and families adopting a holistic focus. This chapter will also enable students to develop and expand their problem-solving skills, as well focusing on the professional values required in a complex healthcare environment. The chapter provides practical skills for both adult and mental health and learning disability nursing students in areas such as performing and recording clinical observations, tips and techniques on maintaining patients' hygiene – e.g. eye care, mouth care – how to use pressure-relieving aids and nutritional assessments.

Chapter 6 Introduction to anatomy and physiology This chapter provides understanding of the structure and function of many of the body's systems and how the human body maintains health; homeostasis is a theme that runs throughout the chapter. The chapter covers the main systems of the body in relation to anatomy and physiology, the content of which will equip student nurses with the necessary knowledge to inform first-year nursing practice and provide the underpinning for progression to qualification.

Chapter 7 Person-centred care: from secondary to primary care The purpose of this chapter is to introduce the student to nursing knowledge and skills required to deliver contemporary adult nursing care in secondary and primary care settings. The chapter enables the student to understand and utilise person-centred approaches to care from ethical, legal and professional perspectives. This chapter builds on Chapter 1's primary care concept and initiatives, such as every contact counts and the 6Cs. In addition, the chapter introduces the student to the use of critical thinking skills in nursing assessment and the delivery of person-centred care. It is expected that this chapter will enable students to merge knowledge, practical ability and professional attitudes in promoting quality, safe patient/client care.

Chapter 8 Understanding pharmacology and introducing medicines management This chapter aims to develop knowledge and understanding of the principles of pharmacology and medicines management with an emphasis on clinical application. It explores and discusses the principles of the pharmacology of groups of drugs commonly used in clinical practice. It considers and evaluates the role and responsibilities of the nurse in relation to the safe administration of medication in clinical practice, including competency with drug calculations that students in the first year of nurse education will need to achieve.

Chapter 9 Death, dying and cultural practices within palliative end-of-life care This chapter aims to develop the students' knowledge and understanding of palliative care and end-of-life issues. It provides the student with an opportunity to explore personal coping strategies and personal beliefs in relation to end-of-life and palliative care issues. Effective communication strategies in relation to end-of-life issues among a diverse population is one of the areas explored to enhance the student's knowledge and skills. It will provide students with an understanding of different cultural practices associated with death and dying.

Chapter 10 Contemporary issues in nursing This chapter focuses on dementia, Alzheimer's disease and delirium. It covers assessment and care management. It begins by introducing the student to the role of patient and family information support in complex care, as well as the role of social care. Dementia is now the number one killer in the UK and most students will encounter a patient with dementia on their placement. It is important that students understand this group of illnesses in the foundation stage of their education that demands much attention of the nurse.

Requirements for the NMC Standards for Pre-registration Nursing Education

Requirements from the NMC Standards

Effective nursing practice requires the nurse to have knowledge and skills, which are outlined in detail in the document Standards of Proficiency for Registered Nurses (NMC, 2018). These Standards are used by educational institutions when planning professional courses. They are grouped into seven 'Platforms', as shown in the box.

Standards of proficiency for registered nurses (NMC, 2018)

Platform 1: Being an accountable professional

Registered nurses act in the best interests of people, putting them first and providing nursing care that is person-centred, safe and compassionate. They act professionally at all times and use their knowledge and experience to make evidence-based decisions

---

about care. They communicate care effectively, are role models for others and are accountable for their actions. Registered nurses continually reflect on their practice, and keep abreast of new and emerging developments in nursing, health and care.

Platform 2: Promoting health and preventing ill health

Registered nurses play a key role in improving and maintaining the mental, physical and behavioural health and well-being of people, families, communities and populations. They support and enable people at all stages of life and in all care settings to make informed choices about how to manage health challenges in order to maximise their quality of life and improve health outcomes. They are actively involved in the prevention of and protection against disease and ill health, and engage in public health, community development and global health agendas, and in the reduction of health inequalities.

Platform 3: Assessing needs and planning care

Registered nurses prioritise the needs of people when assessing and reviewing their mental, physical, cognitive, behavioural, social and spiritual needs. They use information obtained during assessments to identify the priorities and requirements for person-centred and evidence-based nursing interventions and support. They work in partnership with people to develop person-centred care plans that take into account their circumstances, characteristics and preferences.

Platform 4: Providing and evaluating care

Registered nurses take the lead in providing evidence-based, compassionate and safe nursing interventions. They ensure that the care they provide and delegate is person-centred and of a consistently high standard. They support people of all ages in a range of care settings. They work in partnership with people, families and carers to evaluate whether care is effective and the goals of care have been met in line with their wishes, preferences and desired outcomes.

Platform 5: Leading and managing nursing care and working in teams

Registered nurses provide leadership by acting as a role model for best practice in the delivery of nursing care. They are responsible for managing nursing care and are accountable for the appropriate delegation and supervision of care provided by others in the team including lay carers. They play an active and equal role in the interdisciplinary team, collaborating and communicating effectively with a range of colleagues.

Platform 6: Improving safety and quality of care

Registered nurses make a key contribution to the continuous monitoring and quality improvement of care and treatment in order to enhance health outcome and

(Continued)

(Continued)

people's experience of nursing and related care. They assess risks to safety or experience and take appropriate action to manage those, putting the best interests, needs and preferences of people first.

Platform 7: Coordinating care

Registered nurses play a leadership role in coordinating and managing the complex nursing and integrated care needs of people at any stage of their lives, across a range of organisations and settings. They contribute to processes of organisational change through an awareness of local and national policies.

This book draws from these Standards and presents the relevant ones at the beginning of each chapter.

Learning features

Learning from reading text is not always easy. Therefore, to provide variety and to assist with the development of independent learning skills and the application of theory to practice, this book contains activities, case studies, scenarios, further reading, useful websites and other materials to enable you to participate in your own learning. You will need to develop your own study skills and 'learn how to learn' to get the best from the material. The book cannot provide all the answers, but instead provides a framework for your learning.

The activities in the book will help you in particular to make sense of, and learn about, the material being presented. Some activities ask you to reflect on aspects of practice or your experience of it, or the people or situations you encounter. *Reflection* is an essential skill in nursing, and it helps you to understand the world around you and often to identify how things might be improved. Other activities will help you develop key graduate skills such as your ability to *think critically* about a topic in order to challenge received wisdom, or your ability to *research a topic and find appropriate information and evidence,* and to be able to *make decisions* using that evidence in situations that are often difficult and time-pressured. Communication and working as part of a team are core to all nursing practice, and some activities will ask you to carry out *team work activities* or think about your *communication skills* to help develop these. Finally, as a registered nurse, you will be expected to *lead and manage* your own team, case load or area of care, so some activities focus on helping you to build confidence in doing this.

All the activities require you to take a break from reading the text, think through the issues presented and carry out some independent study, possibly using the internet. Where appropriate, there are sample answers presented at the end of each chapter, and these will help you to understand more fully your own reflections and independent study. Remember, academic study will always require independent work; attending lectures will never be enough to be successful on your programme, and these activities will help to deepen your knowledge and understanding of the issues under scrutiny and give you practice at working on your own.

You might want to think about completing these activities as part of your personal development plan (PDP) or portfolio. After completing the activity, write it up in your PDP or portfolio in a section devoted to that particular skill, then look back over time to see how far you are developing. You can also do more of the activities for a key skill that you have identified a weakness in, which will help build your skill and confidence in this area.

As the editor of this book, I hope that you will enjoy using the text in your nursing journey, that it gives you a real-world experience of nursing and contributes positively to your nursing career.

Chapter 1 Professional values and practice

Marie Culloty and Beverly Joshua

NMC Standards of Proficiency for Registered Nurses

Platform 1: Being an accountable professional

Registered nurses act in the best interests of people, putting them first and providing nursing care that is person-centred, safe and compassionate. They act professionally at all times and use their knowledge and experience to make evidence-based decisions about care. They communicate effectively, are role models for others and are accountable for their actions. Registered nurses continually reflect on their practice and keep abreast of new emerging developments in nursing, health and care.

At the point of registration, the registered nurse will be able to:

1.1 understand and act in accordance with The Code (2015): Professional standards of practice and behaviour for nurse midwives and fulfil all registration requirements;

1.2 understand and apply relevant legal, regulatory and governance requirements, policies, and ethical frameworks, including any mandatory reporting duties, to all areas of practice, differentiating where appropriate between the devolved legislatures of the United Kingdom;

1.3 understand and apply the principles of courage, transparency and the professional duty of candour recognising and reporting any situations, behaviours or errors that could result in poor care outcomes;

1.4 demonstrate an understanding of, and the ability to challenge, discriminatory behaviour;

1.6 understand the professional responsibility to adopt a healthy lifestyle to maintain the level of personal fitness and wellbeing required to meet people's needs for mental and physical care;

1.9 understand the need to base all decisions regarding care and interventions on people's needs and preferences, recognising and addressing any personal and external factors that may unduly influence their decisions.

Platform 3: Assessing needs and planning care

Registered nurses prioritise the needs of people when assessing and reviewing their mental, physical, cognitive, behavioural, social and spiritual needs. They use information obtained during assessments to identify the priorities and requirements for person-centred and evidence-based nursing interventions and support. They work in partnership with people to develop person-centred care plans that take into account their circumstances, characteristics and preferences.

3.4 understand and apply a person-centred approach to nursing care, demonstrating shared assessment, planning, decision making and goal setting when working with people, their families, communities and populations of all ages

Chapter aims

After reading this chapter, you will be able to:

- define nursing and identify the characteristics of a profession;
- understand some of the key historical events, organisations and polices in nursing that have shaped contemporary nursing and nurse education;
- understand the role of the professional body – the Nursing and Midwifery Council (NMC) – its functions, the code of practice and how this relates to your clinical practice and your everyday life;
- identify nursing models, and the nursing process.

Introduction

A popular phrase often utilised by healthcare professionals is 'First do no harm', which is often attributed to the Hippocratic Oath taken by doctors who enter the medical profession on completion of their training. Safety is at the heart of all healthcare professionals' work and in all encounters with patients' carers and the general public. The NHS treats up to I million patients every 36 hours (DH, 2005) and employs over a million people. Nurses make up the largest of the groups of healthcare workers with 285,893 employed within the NHS (NHS Digital, 2017). It is essential in the context of modern healthcare that quality and safety are at the heart of caring and practice. In recent years, NHS scandals like that at Mid Staffordshire where hundreds of patients died as result of substandard care and staff failings, have had an impact on the public confidence in the NHS and the image of nursing has also been affected. The subsequent public inquiry chaired by Robert Francis, QC made 290 recommendations calling for more openness, transparency and candour among NHS staff (Francis, 2013). The impact of this report has been immense and far-reaching on all who work within the NHS. Patient safety remains one of the main priorities of a modern health service and is at the heart of good-quality nursing care. The new 2018 Nursing and Midwifery Council Standards place safety and compassion as a key requirement for registrants.

This chapter seeks to identify the professional values and principles that underpin safe, effective, evidence-based care, by defining what nursing is. It will do this by looking at key historical events, including professional registration for nurses and key developments that bring us to current contemporary practice. The chapter starts off with defining nursing, with a brief historical overview of nursing as a profession. This is followed by an overview of the Royal College of Nursing (RCN) and exploring what it means to be a nurse. The roles and functions of the Nursing and Midwifery Council (NMC), together with the standards for practice and pre-registration education, are discussed in this chapter, concluding with the NHS constitution.

Being a nurse carries great responsibility for the patients in your care. The values and principles that guide your actions cover not only your practice, but all aspects of your behaviour, attitude and approach. Unlike all other professions, nursing is unique in its relationship with the patient, as it looks more holistically at the patient's physical, psychological, social and cultural needs. In order to understand nursing, it is necessary to define nursing and related characteristics.

Defining nursing

The word 'nurse' is defined in the *Oxford Dictionary* (2017) as *the practice of caring for the sick and injured*, with the word 'nursing' in Latin meaning *to nourish*. This is, however, a very simplified definition of nurse. It is necessary to look at the term in more detail as applied to the occupation and profession of nursing.

As nursing is a worldwide profession, it is useful to look at how it is defined internationally as indicated by the International Council of Nurses (ICN) whose mission it is to represent nursing worldwide and to advance the profession by influencing health policy. The ICN (2012) defines nursing as encompassing

> *autonomous and collaborative care of individuals of all ages, families, groups and communities, sick or well and in all settings. Nursing includes the care of the ill and end of life care, promotion of health, prevention of illness, and the caring for the disabled and those presenting with mental health. Key nursing roles also includes advocacy, promotion of a safe environment, research, participation in shaping health policy and in patient and health systems management, and education.*

(ICN, 2012, p868)

This broad definition identifies a range of activities, roles and characteristics that nursing is concerned with. Within the United Kingdom (UK), the RCN defines *nursing as the use of clinical judgement in the provision of care to enable people to improve, maintain or recover health to cope with health problems, and to achieve the best possible quality of life whatever their disease or disability until death using six defining characteristics* (RCN, 2014, p3). The six characteristics are:

1. Particular purpose: The purpose is to promote the health of individuals and groups, aiming for healing, growth and development in an attempt to prevent illness, disease and disability. Another purpose is to minimise distress and suffering when people become ill and at the end of life maintain the best possible quality of life thorough nursing care.

2. Particular mode of intervention: This characteristic is concerned with empowering people to achieve, maintain or recover independence. They can do this by using their intellectual, physical and emotional or moral strength. The overall aim is to provide support, identify people's needs and respond to the need both in terms of management, but also in policy development.

3. Particular domain: This characteristic is concerned with understanding the unique response of individuals to disease, illness or disability. Its underlying principle is to understand that these responses may be physiological, psychological, social, spiritual or cultural, and often a combination of one or more. These can be presented in all age groups.

4. Particular focus: This characteristic is person-centred. As a nurse, you will look at the whole person. Here, you consider the entire person not only the condition or an aspect of it.

5. Particular value base: This characteristic focuses on the ethical values, respect and dignity that nursing is based on. It acknowledges that the uniqueness of human beings and that the patient–nurse relationship is a privilege that carries with it responsibility and accountability.

6. Commitment to partnership: This characteristic focuses on working in partnership with patients, carers and others as part of a wider multidisciplinary team. It demonstrates your leadership in delegating and supervising others while remaining accountable for their actions and decisions.

(RCN, 2014, p3)

The above definitions of nursing demonstrate some of the complexity involved in identifying what nursing is and the many domains that it covers. It is not simply a series of tasks that are performed or just a set of skills and knowledge. All nurses carry with them a unique personal concept of what nursing is for them. This might be based on their own experiences of health or caring. It is often difficult to communicate this to others in words, although the desire to help and care for people is a common theme among nurses. Having definitions of nursing is useful in terms of how practitioners view their role and gives us a useful opportunity to reflect on our own values and behaviour. Therefore, values are key elements of nursing as they form the foundation of professional nursing practice and the decisions you make as a developing professional nurse. To help your understanding of values and how they affect your clinical practice, it is worth exploring the meaning of the term 'values' and the concepts related to the development of professionalism in nursing.

The *Oxford Dictionary* defines values as *principles or standards of behaviour and one's judgement of what is important in life*. This may simply be interpreted as a *conviction of what is right, good and desirable and motivates both social and professional behaviour* (Rassin, 2010, p458). In nursing, an example of values is to protect human dignity and be respectful with people. Therefore, your professional values are rooted in your personal values and these are influenced by your family, your culture, your environment, your religious beliefs, as well as ethnic attributes. As a result, the awareness, acquisition and development of your professional values is a gradual process that evolves throughout your personal and professional lifetime (Rassin, 2010).

Professional organisations can be useful in articulating the key principles that underpin nursing and provide us with an identity that we can share and develop to reflect changes in both practice and society. The Royal College of Nursing (RCN) in 2010 identified eight principles of nursing practice that constitute safe and effective nursing care developed in partnership with nurses, patients and the professional regulator (which is the NMC). These principles are identified as:

- Dignity
- Responsibility
- Risk management
- Patient-centred care
- Communication
- Knowledge and skills
- Team working
- Leadership

(RCN, 2010)

Activity 1.1 aims to explore the difference between professional nursing and nursing performed by non-qualified carers.

Activity 1.1   Research and reflection

In 2014, the Royal College of Nursing provided a very useful document, *Defining Nursing*. Please read pages 2–4 from the Useful website link no. 1 at the end of the chapter.

List four things that make a nurse different from a family member undertaking the role.

Write a short definition of what you think nursing is, based on your reading and your own experiences. Identify values that you think are essential to nursing.

An outline answer is provided at the end of the chapter.

Now that you have a better understanding of the characteristics of a nursing professional, in the next section we will look at a brief history of nursing.

Nursing as a profession: a brief history

In order to understand contemporary nursing as a profession today, it is necessary to see how nursing has developed historically. It is also important to look at key organisations and policies that have influenced the development of nursing. During the Middle Ages in Europe, nursing or tending to the sick was primarily the feature of religious orders who dedicated themselves to the service of the infirm. By the 1800s, nurses in England were employed but poorly paid, often working in voluntary or Poor Law infirmaries or, in some cases, in patients' own homes. In addition to paid employment, nurses' work was frequently performed by able-bodied poor people in these institutions. The origins of modern professional nursing in the United Kingdom can be traced back to the early 1860s with Florence Nightingale's return from the Crimean War (1853–6) and the setting up of the first training school for nurses at St Thomas hospital in London (National Archives, n.d.) Other training schools soon followed in different hospitals throughout the UK. This led to an increased growth in training places. The growth in practical nursing assisted with the care of the wounded in the First World War. A voluntary register existed by 1908 as pressure from the British Nurses Association founded in 1887 to seek registration similar to the medical profession. In 1919, the General Nursing Council (GNC) became responsible for professional control, following the Nurses Registration Act providing for the beginnings of modern nursing as we recognise it.

The Registration Act of 1919 provided for a State Nursing Register. This saw the introduction and identification of the minimum level of training required for all nurses to enter the Register. By the mid-1940s, nurse training was extended to include other specialisms, including mental health nursing and the addition of the State Enrolled Nurses to the registry. Enrolled nursing was orientated towards more practical nursing, with less managerial responsibility. The training was for two years, in comparison to the State Registered Nurses' training, which was for three years. The creation of the NHS in the late 1940s witnessed more changes in healthcare provision and an increase in the numbers of nurses and training places. By 1951, male nurses had joined the main nursing register which, up to this point, had been a female-dominant occupation. Most training was conducted in Schools of Nursing affiliated to hospitals and nurse teachers were pre-dominantly trained nurses who had completed recognised training courses to become nurse tutors. Courses followed an apprentice-style training, with student nurses being paid as employees of the hospital who generally lived in hospital accommodation for some period of their training if they required it. At the end of the training period and having passed clinical assessments on wards, students sat the state exam paper and, on successful attainment, were eligible to register as a State Registered Nurse (SRN) or State Enrolled Nurse (SEN). This later became the Registered General Nurse (RGN) qualification. At most schools of nursing, the newly qualified nurses wore a badge with the coat of arms of their hospital, school or university.

By the 1970s, nurses were undertaking a variety of roles in clinical practice. The development of specialisms in medicine and surgery was also mirrored in nursing role development – for example, the role of pain specialist nurse. Post-registration courses approved by the English National Board became the main route for nurses to specialise and diversify their career pathway. This meant that employment prospects had expanded greatly by the 1980s. In 1983, the General Nursing Council (GNC) was replaced by the United Central Council for Nursing, Midwifery and Health Visiting (UKCC), which was responsible for registration, and the national Boards for Nursing, which were responsible for training, education and the assessment of all nurses. In 1986, the newly formed UKCC launched Project 2000 – a wide-ranging reform of nurse education aimed at improving the academic standing of the curriculum from certifi-cate level to diploma level, and moving away from the former apprenticeship style to higher education-based training (Allen, 2009).

In 1997, the government set out the direction to modernise the NHS and improve the health of the population in its key document *The New NHS: Modern, Dependable.* Key to this change was the desire to change nurse training to take account of the range of clinical skills needed at the point of registration and to meet the challenges of increas-ing technology and patient expectations. *Making a difference: Strengthening the Nursing, Midwifery and Health Visiting Contribution to Health and Healthcare* (DH, 1999) set out the new model of nurse education which was designed to improve career opportunities, access to nursing and provide a framework for post-registration education. This was done in order to support the expanding roles and specialist areas of practice, and to enable a nurse to develop a clinical career pathway from healthcare assistant to reg-istered nurse to consultant or expert nurse positions in clinical practice. This career progression was achieved by demonstrating competence and advanced skills. In the late 1990s, the differentiation between advanced practice and specialist practice was more complete, and the UKCC defined advance practice as not being an

> *additional layer of practice to be superimposed on specialist nursing practice. It is, rather, a description of an important sphere of professional practice which is concerned with the continuing development of the professions in the interest of patients, clients and health services.*

(UKCC, 1994)

By the late 1990s nurse training was transformed by the introduction of Project 2000.

The Nursing and Midwifery Council (NMC) replaced the UKCC in April 2002 and also took over the quality assurance of nurse education formally undertaken by the English National Board. The Nursing and Midwifery Council provides institutions with the standards for pre-registration training that all nursing programmes and courses need to meet and against which institutions providing these courses will be approved and monitored.

The 1990s onwards saw a growth and expansion of the roles of nurses, who took on duties that had previously been performed by medical staff. Many of these early duties and roles involved in-house training and included duties like venepuncture and cannulation. Supported by the RCN, many clinical specialist areas developed specialist nurse roles. These roles included areas like oncology or diabetes, and, as a result, courses and future study were developed by education providers to meet the needs of nurses wanting to specialise in these areas. Many of the early courses were at a minimum of degree level. By 2002, nurses were able to prescribe medications and there was a requirement by the profession and employers that nurses used evidence in their practice. This resulted in the Royal College of Nursing vote in 2008 to seek an all-graduate profession (RCN, 2009). By 2006, Advanced Nurse Practitioner role descriptions were more clearly defined to incorporate a number of key advanced skills, competence and knowledge that practitioners need to demonstrate and were recordable by the NMC. In 2011, the first wave of graduate-only education came into place and by 2012, all students were commencing degree-only courses, leading to registration.

The image and identity of nursing is linked to both its history and to the role of women in society and the workplace. Over recent decades, nursing image and identity has been shaped by the policy, social, cultural and media portal of nursing. Egenes (2017) holds the view that the lack of critical historical awareness can view the past as a golden age of nursing. This view can fail to consider the issues and concerns raised in the past – for example, the issues of the standards of care that were evident in the 1960s and early 1970s. Typical stereotypes, including that of handmaiden, angel and sex object, often requiring manual working and performing tasks that involve bodily fluids, have continued, partly resulting from the historical idea of what nurses do, to the media portal of nurses. Some would argue that it is these images that have impacted on the failure to recruit well-educated potential candidates to nursing, and that more realistic images of nursing are needed to alter people's and society's perceptions (Ferns and Chojnacka, 2005).

How is nurse education different in Europe?

Most European countries have a generic curriculum in that students are educated to look after children, adult and mental health patients. This is unlike the United Kingdom, which has four separate strands of specialist fields, as well as a separate midwifery strand, all of which lead to registration at degree or baccalaureate level and with varying lengths of three- to four-year courses.

Now that you have read a little about how nursing as a profession developed, take a look at Activity 1.2 in order to develop your understanding.

Activity 1.2   Reflection

Below is a list of possible characteristics necessary for a professional qualification. Circle those you believe are correct.

- There is a set curriculum to study for the professional qualification.
- The profession has a self-regulation.
- Professional qualification allows one to be autonomous.
- A profession has as an ethical code to guide practice.
- A profession has a legal basis by which they practise.
- A profession has a set minimum level of education.
- A profession has a body of knowledge.
- Professional people are accountable for their actions.
- Professionals wear an identifiable uniform.
- Professionals are required to maintain confidentiality.

In the following list of occupations, circle those you believe meet the characteristics of a profession. Give reasons for your choices:

teacher, solicitor, beautician, dentist, veterinary surgeon, bank manager, chartered accountant, social worker, actor, hairdresser, nail technician.

An outline answer is provided at the end of the chapter.

Having considered what it means to be a professional person, we now look at the nursing profession in particular.

The Royal College of Nursing: its role and function in nursing

The College of Nursing Ltd was originally a professional organisation for trained nurses formed in 1916 with just 34 members. Later, in 1977, it became a trade union and nursing organisation with the central aim of providing support, representing, promoting excellence and contribute to shaping health policies. It received its royal charter in 1928 and became the Royal College of Nursing with the Queen as its patron. Since its inception, it has included within its members registered nurses; students were admitted in 1968 and in 2001 healthcare assistants were admitted (RCN, 2016). Historically, the

RCN has utilised its membership to shape its direction and inform its policies through consultation and debate among its members. The RCN has a wide stewardship that provides professional guidance and support to its members as part of its trade union role. As a student nurse or new graduate, being a member of a trade union can provide you with support in the event of any fitness to practise allegation being raised. There are many other trade unions that also provide this service and offer support and guidance. The students' union on campus can also provide you with support, but be aware that in paid employment it can be useful to have support that is conversant with roles and responsibilities of nurses within healthcare environments and the boundaries that you are expected to work within.

The next activity is designed to make you reflect on the qualities that you expect from a nurse.

Activity 1.3 Reflection

What qualities do you think a professional nurse should have? From the list below, pick six to eight words that you think best describe a professional nurse. You might want to place them in order of preference from 1 to 8:

kindness, respectful, caring, resilient, helpful, non-judgemental, hardworking, dignified, selfless, knowledgeable, aware of one's own limitations, confident, trustworthy, honest, creative, polite, compassionate.

An outline answer is provided at the end of the chapter.

Now that you are more familiar with the qualities expected from a nurse, and that these may not always be professional characteristics, let us now consider what is expected of the modern professional nurse.

Nursing as a profession

As can be seen from the history of nursing, the early years were predominantly hospital and practical based and seen as a vocation, with nurses providing a service to the wider community. The creation of schools of nursing provided more of an apprentice-style training than its modern counterparts. However, the push to professionalism can clearly be seen even in the early twentieth century, and the creation of the Nurses Registration Act in 1919 initiated the starting point in the drive for nursing to gain professional status and to be viewed by other professions in the same light. The creation of a regulatory body with the power to enforce standards for the education of nurses, the provision of a code of conduct and a mechanism for ensuring fitness to practise have all assisted with the move to increase professionalism. The creation of a graduate-level qualification has also ensured that nursing in terms of educational attainment matches that of fellow medical and allied health professionals.

What does it mean to be a professional?

You are a member of an occupational group of people who share a similar set of values, knowledge and skills that are recognised by the wider society as belonging to the nursing profession. To meet this requirement, you will need to meet the standards of education, and skills and knowledge acquisition and set of proficiencies required at the point of registration as identified by the NMC. As a professional nurse, you will become responsible for your actions and decisions you make, and you will be held to account for these by your regulator. As a result, there are clear expectations of you in terms of your actions, by your colleagues and the general public. The expected norm is that you will always act in the best interest of your patient at all situations as you need to be able to justify your decisions, actions and omissions, even if you were instructed by another professional (NMC, 2015). In practice, this means that when nursing patients:

- you should know why you're doing it;
- you should have been properly trained and assessed as being competent to do it;
- you should be doing it as part of an agreed plan of care for the patient/client.

(RCN, 2015)

Development towards being a professional starts from the moment of application to undertake a nursing programme of study by ensuring that students and prospective nurses have the right attributes and values that will help them to meet the needs of patients. These values are common to many healthcare professions and are commonly referred to as the 6Cs of nursing, introduced by the then Chief Nursing Officer for England, Jane Cummings, in 2012 as part of the Compassion in Practice policy document. The vision and strategy for nurses, midwives and healthcare staff, the 6Cs identifies six areas of action to support professionals and care staff to deliver excellent care and is underpinned by six fundamental values.

The 6Cs of nursing are:

- **Compassion**: Describes the care administered being based on empathy, dignity and respect.
- **Competence**: Indicates that all care-givers must have the ability to understand the patient's needs, and have the clinical and technical knowledge to deliver effective evidenced-based care.
- **Care**: This is the foundation of the care-giver's role and helps improve the patient's health. People in receipt of care expect to be given the right treatment at all times.

- **Communication:** This is essential for optimum care to be delivered, incorporates active listening skills and is crucial for effective team involvement within the care-giving environment.
- **Courage:** Having courage ensures that care-givers always choose to do the right action for those in their care. It also gives them the personal strength to speak up or report issues that concern them, so that improved actions can be implemented.
- **Commitment:** Being committed is the foundation of the care-giver's role and allows them to embrace new and innovative ways in order that the patient's experience and the healthcare challenges are met.

(DH, 2012)

These 6Cs have underpinned not only recruitment to nursing courses but also to NHS positions.

Nursing and Midwifery Council (NMC): role and function

The Health Act 1999 provided the legislation that allowed for regulation of the nursing profession. The Nursing and Midwifery Order 2001 (the Order) is, in fact, a series of orders made by the Privy Council and the United Kingdom Central Council for Nursing, Midwifery and Health Visiting (UKCC), which came into effect on 1 April 2002. The Order established the NMC, creating its structure, function and activities, and set its primary purpose of protecting the public. Among the series of orders and rules are specific orders relating to parts of the register and protected titles that only nurses on that part of the register can use.

Role of the NMC

The NMC is responsible for regulating nurses and midwives in England, Wales, Scotland and Northern Ireland. It exists to protect the public and to regulate the profession by:

- setting standards for education, training, conduct and performance;
- ensuring that nurses and midwives keep their skills and knowledge up to date and uphold the professional standards expected, ensuring that nurses renew their registration every year and revalidate every three years, providing evidence of their updating and professional development;
- providing, as a regulator, clear and transparent processes to investigate and determine the outcome following panel hearings, when nurses fall short of the required standards;

- providing mechanisms for both employers and members of the public to raise concern about any nurse's practice;
- maintaining a register of nurses and midwives who are allowed to practise in the UK, and provide employers and the general public to check this register to ensure that practitioners are allowed to practise.

The NMC's professional standards for practice: code of practice

All healthcare professionals have their own code of conduct setting out the standards of ethical behaviour owed by members of each profession. The NMC's code of conduct, also referred to as *The Code*, first published in 2008 and revised in 2015, outlines the professional standards that nurses and midwives must uphold in order to be registered to practise in the UK. The code of practice draws on earlier codes and guidelines provided by its predecessor, the UKCC, which set out the guidelines in 1983. The current NMC *Code* of 2015 was updated to reflect the changing roles and expectations of nurses and midwives in the way they work and live (NMC, 2015).

The Code is structured around four main themes:

- prioritising people;
- practising effectively;
- preserving safety;
- promoting professionalism and trust.

The Code provides assurances about the expected standards of care and behaviour that patients can expect from nurses. Employers also can utilise the *Code* to determine the suitability of a nurse to practise if there are concerns about them. The *Code* provides the basis by which the NMC assesses a nurse or midwife who is referred to them where a concern has been raised. The following case study and associated activity allows you to explore this in more detail.

Case study: Barry

Following an NMC's fitness to practise panel hearing in 2013, a qualified nurse, Barry White (a fictitious name) was banned from working for six months. The reason for this was that he posted a series of inappropriate comments and pictures on Facebook.

Barry made derogatory comments that ran to 45 pages about his workplace and jobs, also referring to other colleagues and students by inappropriate terms. Staff nurse Barry White named the place of work on the social media site. Postings also referred to drinking and the post contained sexual references. This also included a picture of a colleague on a bedpan. In the defence given, Barry suggested that it was only viewed by his personal friends.

The above case study highlights the issue of social media and its use. It explores the problem that as a practitioner someone might assume that a posting is only seen by friends when it is, in fact, accessible to the public. As a nurse practitioner, we need to understand that this can undermine public confidence in the nursing profession and that it breaches NMC guidelines. Use the activity below to explore your own thoughts around professionalism.

Activity 1.4   Research and reflection

Please go to the Useful websites section at the end of the chapter, link no. 2, to complete this activity. These refer to any social media site.

Thinking about professionalism, show which behaviour you think is profes-sional or unprofessional in the six listed below by circling Yes/No and may result in difficulties with being registered as a qualified nurse. Use the terms A–E, where A represents Dishonest, B represents Criminal, C represents Fraudulent, D represents Breach of confidentiality and E represents None of these. Circle the letter which you think most closely reflects the behaviour.

1. Shouting at a colleague   Yes/No (A), (B), (C), (D), (E)

2. Using Facebook to discuss a patient's conditions with your friends

        Yes/No (A), (B), (C), (D), (E)

3. Taking equipment for your first-aid box from the ward

        Yes/No (A), (B), (C), (D), (E)

4. Eating a patient's food   Yes/No (A), (B), (C), (D), (E)

5. Using a family member's travel documents to

    obtain cheap travel   Yes/No   (A), (B), (C), (D), (E)

6. Incurring a parking fine   Yes/No   (A), (B), (C), (D), (E)

An outline answer is available at the end of the chapter.

As a student nurse, you need to be aware that your behaviour and the image you pro-ject both at work and outside of work can affect the public's perception of nursing. Being aware of the boundaries is an important aspect of your development as a profes-sional. In nursing, you come in contact with people who are at their most vulnerable and behaving in a professional, caring and compassionate manner will help you gain trust and respect from the patient's carers and family members. It is important to judge the difference between being friendly and helpful, and being too familiar. Revealing too much personal information may mean that you become over-familiar. As a result, you could place yourself and the patient in a difficult position and compromise your professional relationship. Social media and its use can also prove problematic. You need to know the boundaries of what you can upload. Remember that social media can be viewed by other people, so making inappropriate comments about patients, colleagues or work places may lead to a breach in confidentiality.

The case study below is designed to allow you to explore a situation on professional relationships and maintaining professional boundaries.

Case study: Charlotte

Charlotte is a student nurse and a friend of yours. Both of you are allocated to the same ward. She tells you that she is very fond of Jamal, who is a patient with a sporting injury. Charlotte confided in you that although Jamal is very flirtatious with all the nurses, he has apparently confessed to being in love with her. Charlotte says that she thinks that the feeling is mutual. You notice that Charlotte has requested to be allocated to Jamal's cubicle to assist him with his personal hygiene.

Activity 1.5 asks you to explore this case study in more detail.

Activity 1.5   Critical thinking

1.   Consider your response when being told of the situation.
2.   What actions would you take?
3.   Provide rationale for your decisions.

An outline answer is provided at the end of the chapter.

The case study above highlights the importance of maintaining professional relationships and boundaries. It explores a situational issue of developing romantic interests in patients who are entrusted to your care. The change in the platonic nurse–patient relationship does impact on the care that nurses administer to patients. Such changes in the nurse–patient dynamic will affect the care given to other patients and prevent you from treating all patients as equals.

The NMC's professional standards for pre-registration education

Another important role of the NMC, as already indicated, is to provide the standards for pre-registration courses and programmes for all fields of nursing that institutions (both higher education and private providers) must meet in order to prepare nurses for registration. So, for example, the course you are already on will have very specific requirements about the proficiencies you will need to achieve at the point of registration, and the number of practical hours and theory hours that the course must contain to be compliant with the NMC's directives. There are also the standards that the NMC can use to monitor the quality of education and compliance. The 2004 standards of proficiency for pre-registration nurse education was replaced in 2010 by the standards for pre-registration nurse education, taking into account major policies such as Modernising Nursing Careers (DH, 2006). These standards have now been replaced by the latest standards published in 2018 (NMC, 2018).

Nursing and the NHS Constitution

Since the introduction of the NHS in 1948, nurses' roles have changed and adapted to meet new challenges posed by improvements in science and technology, resulting in new treatments, and in changes in how and where care is delivered. However, the founding principles of the NHS are based on three core principles: that it meets the needs of everyone, that it is free at the point of delivery, and that it is based on clinical need, not the ability to pay. In March 2011, the Department of Health published the NHS Constitution for England, updated in October 2015, which sets out the guiding principles of the NHS and the rights of NHS patients and staff who work in the NHS (DH, 2015).

The constitution provides seven key principles that guide the NHS in all that it does.

- The constitution provides a comprehensive service, available to all.
- The constitution makes clear that access to NHS services is based on clinical need, not on an individual's ability to pay.
- The constitution empowers health care workers to aspire to the highest standards of excellence and professionalism.
- The constitution makes clear that all patients should be at the heart of everything the NHS does.
- The constitution recommends that all health care staff work across organisational boundaries.
- Through the constitution, all health care workers are committed to providing the best value for taxpayers' money.
- Through the constitution, all health care workers are accountable to the public, communities and patients that it serves.

The constitution also sets out the values expected of all who provide care and were developed in partnership with staff and patients. These values apply to every employee in the NHS, no matter their position. This position can be either in direct care – that is, looking after and caring for their patients and families – or it could also be in supporting non-clinical or any provider – that is, those not responsible for patient care or others who may be involved in providing a care service, working in partnership with the NHS to deliver care.

The values set out by the constitution include:

* working together for patients' optimum health;
* showing respect and dignity at all times;
* making a commitment to quality care;
* demonstrating compassion in all care situations;
* working towards improving the lives of the people we care for;
* ensuring that every contact you make counts.

(DH, 2015)

In addition, the constitution makes clear the rights and responsibilities of patients and the public, as well as the rights and responsibilities of staff. The activity below will help you to identify the responsibilities of nurses set within the context of the values of the NHS.

Activity 1.6 Research and reflection

In this activity, we would like you to go to the Useful websites section at the end of the chapter, link no. 3, which will take you to the Department of Health site and look at the NHS Constitution.

After reading the NHS Constitution online, can you identify the nurse's responsibility to patients and the public, and to fellow colleagues?

How might you ensure that you meet these?

An outline answer is provided at the end of the chapter.

Having considered the rights and responsibilities for both nurses, their patients and the public, we now turn to considering models of nursing care.

The evolution of models of nursing care

Traditionally, the theory and practice of nursing was heavily influenced by the aims of medicine (McEwen and Wills, 2018). The medical model dominated early nurse curricula which focused primarily on the doctor determining a diagnosis. This diagnosis was based on the patient's presenting symptoms, prescribing the treatment with the intention of curing the disease. As the nursing profession developed, concerns were raised about the suitability of the medical model in its ability to guide the holistic needs of patients. Holistic needs include the emotional and relationship needs that have an impact on a patient's well-being. The medical model to a greater extent ignored these needs. Nursing curricula in the 1960s was influenced by the development of models of care that had originated in the USA. Nursing models were developed to define the beliefs, values and goals of nursing, as well as the knowledge and skills needed to practise nursing. This shift allowed for a philosophical change and professional status attainment by embracing an alternative to the medical model. Nursing models are, therefore, frameworks that guide nurses' practice and education, and included the following three components.

- A set of beliefs and values.
- The goal that the nurse is attempting to achieve.
- The knowledge and skills that nurses require to practise.

Essentially, all nursing models focus on the following concepts in varying degrees.

- Person – the recipient of the nursing care.
- Health – the condition, either wellness or illness of the recipient of the care.
- Environment – the recipient's specific surroundings.
- Nursing – actions carried out by nurses on behalf of or with the recipient.

In the 1970s, there was a shift to a problem-solving approach to nursing care, and the nursing process model, proposed by Yura and Walsh (1973), was introduced. This model was embedded with values, beliefs and theories of care, comprising a four-stage problem-solving focus (Melin-Johansson et al., 2017). It resulted in the emergence of the concept of a nursing diagnosis. It was also recognised as a *decision-making approach that promoted critical thinking* (Yildirim and Özkahraman, 2011, p261) when administering nursing care. The model commenced with an *assessment,* and involved the collection of information from the patient and their family/carers about their presenting condition and related problems. The *planning* stage followed thereafter and interventions that could resolve the patient's presenting symptoms were identified. The *implementation* phase is then undertaken where care is delivered based on the needs of the patient and the seriousness of the identified problems. The crucial aspect of the nursing process after a thorough assessment of the patient's concerns is the evaluation to assess if the care that was delivered actually achieved the desired outcome. However, as this linear problem-solving technique lacked any reflective component on how clinical decisions were made, it was deemed inadequate, especially by experienced nurses (Melin-Johansson et al., 2017).

In the late 1980s, the Integrated Care Pathway (ICP) was adopted in the UK healthcare system following its development in Boston, USA, in 1985. ICPs are structured tools that incorporate healthcare guidelines, protocols, and evidenced-based, best practice into everyday use for individual patients in the healthcare system. The ICP reflects a patient-centred, multidisciplinary, multiagency approach to each patient's care journey from the peripheral care environment – for example, from the primary care setting, to the hospital admission, to acute care, then progressing to rehabilitation and discharge back to the primary care, if needed. Therefore, the ICPs multidisciplinary/multiagency interlinking allows for the crossing of professional and organisational boundaries, and ensures that the holistic provision of care constructs a unique journey for each individual patient according to their needs, based on professional judgement. The ICP is also an outcome-focused approach with identified standards that need to be achieved as the patient progresses through their care journey. Failure to achieve a key milestone is recorded as a variance in outcomes and professionals, who contribute to the care, and are encouraged to exercise clinical judgement in revising and improving the ICP.

In the 1990s, the Activities of Daily Living (ADLs), also known as the Roper–Logan–Tierney Model for Nursing (Roper et al., 2000) gained widespread popularity in British nursing. Nurses were taught to use the model when assessing how patients' illnesses, injuries or admission to a hospital affected their lives. The ADLs included assessing the patient/client in relation to the following:

- maintaining a safe environment;
- eating and drinking;
- mobilisation;
- communication;
- washing and dressing;
- working and playing;
- breathing;
- controlling temperature;
- sleeping;
- expressing sexuality;
- death and dying;
- elimination.

The findings were then categorised into activities of living, which led to the implementation of interventions to support independence in the areas that the patient might find difficult to undertake on their own. This model encouraged nurses to decide on the interventions that needed to be in place to increase the patient's independence. It also encouraged the ongoing assessment of support that was needed for the patient to remain independent. By measuring the dependence–independence continuum along the patient's lifespan, nurses determined whether the patient was improving or deteriorating. These assessments allowed for the patient's care to be revised, based on the presenting evidence.

Nursing models were positively endorsed in the UK, despite being rooted in other disciplines, in particular medicine, and having initially evolved from an American foundation, with considerable criticisms. However, despite such critique and scrutiny, nursing models have led the way to the current person-centred nursing model being advocated by the NMC (2017) and being included in nursing curricula.

1.14 Provide and promote non-discriminatory, person-centred and sensitive care at all times, reflecting on people's values and beliefs, diverse backgrounds, cultural characteristics, language requirements, needs and preferences, taking account of any need for adjustments

(p9)

The NMC (2017) further defines this person-centred model to nursing as:

an approach where the person is sat the centre of the decision making processes and the design of their care needs, their nursing care and treatment plan.

(p36)

Therefore, all caregivers are required to use a person-centred approach when caring for patients. By adopting this multidimensional model, the patient is in the centre of all decisions made about their needs, their nursing care and treatment plan, and their diversity, culture, religion, spirituality, sexuality, gender, age and disability are also considered. Patients' care is individualised and care options are offered and negotiated through the patient, nurse and multidisciplinary relationship. Using a person-centred model helps to ensure that care provided is accessible, responsive and flexible to meet the diverse needs and preferences of people living in the community. This model's main goal is to allow individuals to remain independent for as long as possible.

Having gained an understanding of nursing models, consider using a person-centred approach in the case study and activity below.

Case study: Mrs Mohammed

Mrs Mohammed is 65 years old. She is admitted to the day-care Surgical Unit for an invasive bladder investigation after complaining of prolonged lower abdominal pain and haematuria. Mrs Mohammed is accompanied by her articulate daughter who seems quite bossy and overbearing. Unlike her daughter, Mrs Mohammed speaks very little English. While admitting Mrs Mohammed, you notice that she is reading the local English newspaper and discussing the article with her daughter. Following the procedure, Mrs Mohammed is diagnosed with terminal cancer of the bladder. Mrs Mohammed then asks you about the outcome of the procedure. However, Mrs Mohammed's daughter calls you aside and tells you that her mother should not be informed of the diagnosis as she would not understand nor cope with the situation. You notice that Mrs Mohammed looks anxious when her daughter and you are speaking.

Activity 1.7   Reflection

As a developing professional who adopts a person-centred approach to care, read the above patient case study and identify the issues regarding Mrs Mohammed's daughter's request.

1. How would you respond to the daughter's request?

2. How would you respond to Mrs Mohammed's request about the outcome of the procedure?

(Continued)

27

(Continued)

3. Consider how withholding information affects the care and treatment the patient receives.

4. Identify the elements of *The Code* that you would use to support your responses.

An outline answer is provided at the end of the chapter.

Having applied a patient-centred nursing model when interacting with patients and their families in situations of uncertainty, referring to and using the NMC's *Code* as a frame of reference will guide your responses and your practice.

The key aim of nursing models was to develop a knowledge base that would make nursing unique from other healthcare-related disciplines, especially medicine. The inception of models for delivering nursing care was to encourage the development of further nursing theories that could be generated, tested and included into the profession's knowledge base. The introduction and use of nursing models represented a significant stage in the development of nursing theory and nursing as a discipline. As the nursing profession continues to develop in the context of a contemporary healthcare environment, delivering integrated, person-centred care will involve co-ordinating care. The combined effect of health and social care systems and services need to work seamlessly with other healthcare professionals – for example, physiotherapists and occupational therapists in assisting with patient rehabilitation. Through such evolutionary changes to the delivery of care, the core principles of nursing models are to acknowledge the value of the person as a human being and their uniqueness as an individual. This will allow the person/patient/client to be seen as a 'whole' as opposed to just concentrating on their presenting health problem.

Chapter summary

This chapter has provided a brief overview of the development of nursing from an apprenticeship-style training to the current all-graduate courses. It has mapped key events in the history of nursing and how nursing has evolved over time to meet the changing needs of the population, and to meet the challenges of improvements in technology and treatment that have shaped the NHS since its beginnings. It outlines the main policy drivers that have had an impact on nursing, and how roles and responsibilities have changed since registration in 1919. The role of the NMC as the professional regulator in terms of standards and fitness to practise and the code of conduct provides every nurse with the underpinning expectations of all nurses. The qualities and values of nursing and the NHS have been identified. The chapter closes with the inclusion of nursing models within the UK healthcare and nurse education context.

Activities: Brief outline answers

Activity 1.1   Research and reflection (p12)

Four things that make a nurse different from a family member undertaking the role.

1. The ability to assess and use your clinical judgement to determine the needs of the unwell person.

2. In-depth knowledge of disease process and treatments.

3. Accountability for the actions and decisions you make, which could have legal implications and an impact on your ability to remain on the nursing register.

4. A professional relationship based on respect and non-judgemental approach rather than a personal relationship.

Although it is true to say that you don't need to be a nurse to care for a person, a nurse has the knowledge, skills and competence to assess the individual needs of a patient and to deliver care in a compassionate and kind, non-judgemental way. Clinical decisions can then be made so that you are accountable for your actions.

Nursing is concerned with caring for ill or injured people in a compassionate manner, utilising a range of knowledge, skills and competence in restoring health, preventing harm and enabling patients to achieve the best quality of life what ever their disease or disability until death.

Activity 1.2   Reflection (p16)

Professions follow a set curriculum that includes a body of knowledge which is guided by an ethical code, leading to a recognised qualification. A profession has a legal basis, is self-regulating, practitioners are autonomous, are accountable and must ensure confidentiality.

Other professionals include: teacher, solicitor, dentist, bank manager, chartered accountant, veterinary surgeon and social worker.

Hairdresser, nail technician, actor – although these professions require skills, training and education, they do not share the same characteristics as those identified above.

Activity 1.3   Reflection (p17)

Caring, compassionate, respectful, non-judgemental, knowledgeable, aware of one's own limitations, honest, resilient and confident.

All of the above are qualities that one would expect in a nurse at the point of registration. Some of the others are also qualities that are equally valued in nursing, and a team that has a good variety and diversity of qualities can be an asset to an organisation. Creativity allows for innovation; hardworking is valued by colleagues. Polite and dignified are qualities that are useful in dealing with the public and can be a valuable asset in any nursing situation. Acting with kindness and selflessness is a trait that is much admired by all patients.

Activity 1.4   Research and reflection (p21)

Please go to the Useful websites section, link no. 2, to complete this activity. Please note that these refer to any social media site.

1. Shouting at a colleague   Yes (E)

2. Using Facebook to discuss a patient's conditions with your friends   Yes (D)

3. Taking equipment for your first aid box from the ward   Yes (A), (B), (C)

4. Eating a patient's food   Yes (A), (B) (B because it can constitute stealing)

5. Using a family member's travel documents to obtain cheap travel   Yes (A), (B), (C), (D)

6. Incurring a parking fine   Yes (E) (you should declare this to your course director as it involves breaking the law)

Activity 1.5   Critical thinking (p22)

As Charlotte's friend, you should attempt to speak to her about the crossing of professional boundaries with a patient. Charlotte needs to be aware that her romantic feelings for Jamal will affect the decisions as a student nurse caring for a patient. It may result in her favouring Jamal over the other patients in her care. In doing so, she would be breaching the professional nursing attributes of treating all patients as equals. Should Charlotte remain adamant, without breaching confidentiality, you may consider seeking support on how to handle this situation from your personal tutor or clinical mentor.

Your rationale will be founded on demonstrating personal integrity and being trusted to act responsibly with patients and all those entrusted to our care. Ethical principles state that we have to treat all individuals fairly and equitably. Therefore, being romantically involved with a patient compromises our ability to treat all patients as equals. We will be biased in the attention and care we administer to the patient we like and favour. It is essential that as developing professionals, we need to be able to separate our personal feelings in order that at all times we demonstrate our good character as identified in *The Code*.

Activity 1.6   Research and reflection (p24)

Right to:

* receive NHS services free of charge;
* access NHS services;
* receive care and treatment appropriate to the patient;
* be treated with a professional standard of care;
* be treated in a clean, safe, secure and suitable environment;
* receive suitable food;
* be treated with dignity and respect, and protected from harm;
* privacy and confidentiality;
* accept professional accountability and maintain standards of professional practice;
* take reasonable care of health and safety at work for you and your team;
* not discriminate against patients or staff and adhere to equal opportunities;
* act in accordance with your employment contact;
* be honest and truthful in carrying out your role;
* provide safe care;
* follow all standards of professional practice;
* stay up to date in your training.

Activity 1.7   Reflection (p27)

Respect the patient's right to know their diagnosis. Tactfully inform relatives that the patient has a right to her personal information including the diagnosis, outcome of the procedure. Therefore, advocate on the patient's behalf. Offer other pastoral supportive measures – e.g. call for a religious leader, or arrange for the patient and family to be visited by hospital-based oncology support group.

Practice guided by the *Code*.

Act in the best interests of the patient. To achieve this you must:

* balance the need to act in the best interests of people at all times with the requirement to respect a person's right to accept or refuse treatment;

- make sure that you get properly informed consent and document it before carrying out any action;
- keep to all relevant laws about mental capacity that apply in the country in which you are practising, and make sure that the rights and best interests of those who lack capacity are still at the centre of the decision-making process;
- tell colleagues, your manager and the person receiving care if you have a conscientious objection to a particular procedure, and arrange for a suitably qualified colleague to take over responsibility for that person's care.

Communicate clearly. To achieve this, you must:

- use terms that people in your care, colleagues and the public can understand;
- take reasonable steps to meet people's language and communication needs, providing, wherever possible, assistance to those who need help to communicate their own or other people's needs;
- use a range of verbal and non-verbal communication methods, and consider cultural sensitivities, to better understand and respond to people's personal and health needs;
- check people's understanding from time to time to keep misunderstanding or mistakes to a minimum;
- be able to communicate clearly and effectively in English.

Recognise and work within your competence. To achieve this, you must:

- accurately assess signs of normal or worsening physical and mental health in the person receiving care;
- make a timely and appropriate referral to another practitioner when it is in the best interests of the individual needing any action, care or treatment;
- ask for help from a suitably qualified and experienced healthcare professional to carry out any action or procedure that is beyond the limits of your competence;
- take account of your own personal safety as well as the safety of people in your care;
- complete the necessary training before carrying out a new role.

Further reading

Griffith, R and Tengnah, C (2014) *Transforming Nursing Practice: Law and Professional Issues in Nursing* (3rd edn). London: SAGE.

This text provides information on professional accountability and the patient's right to decide on treatment, and includes numerous practice-based case studies and examples.

Hall, C and Ritchie, D (2013) *Transforming Nursing Practice: What is Nursing?* (3rd edn). London: SAGE.

This text advances thinking on the defining features of nursing and using a case study approach, expands on what it is to be a professional nurse.

Useful websites

1. Royal College of Nursing (2015) First Steps. London: Royal College of Nursing: **https:// rcni.com/hosted-content/rcn/first-steps/accountability**

This clearly written document provides understanding on what makes nursing a unique profession and is helpful for all new nurses.

2. Nursing and Midwifery Council guidance on using social media: **www.nmc.org.uk/ globalassets/sitedocuments/nmc-publications/social-media-guidance.pdf**

This clearly written document provides guidance on using social media and is helpful to all student and qualified nurses.

3. National Health Service Constitution (2015): **www.gov.uk/government/uploads/system/ uploads/attachment_data/file/480482/NHS_Constitution_WEB.pdf**

4. Department of Health (1999) Making a Difference: Strengthening the Nursing, Midwifery and Health Visiting: **http://webarchive.nationalarchives.gov.uk/20120524072447/http:// www.dh.gov.uk/prod_consum_dh/groups/dh_digitalassets/@dh/@en/documents/ digitalasset/dh_4074704.pdf**

5. Department of Health (2006) Modernising Nursing Careers: Setting the Direction: **www. nursingleadership.org.uk/publications/settingthedirection.pdf**

6. Department of Health (2012) Compassion in Practice: Nursing, Midwifery and Care Staff: Our Vision and Strategy, Gateway reference 18479, London (p13): **http://webarchive. nationalarchives.gov.uk/20120524072447/http://www.dh.gov.uk/prod_consum_dh/ groups/dh_digitalassets/@dh/@en/documents/digitalasset/dh_4074704.pdf**

7. Health Education England, Clinical Academic Careers Framework: A framework for optimising clinical academic careers across healthcare professions: **www.hee.nhs.uk/sites/ default/files/documents/HEE_Clinical_Academic_Careers_Framework.pdf**

8. National Health Service (2017) Draft Standards for Education: **www.nmc.org.uk/ globalassets/sitedocuments/edcons/ec6-draft-standards-for-education-and-training-annexe-1-requirements-for-learning-and-assessment**

9. Nursing and Midwifery Council (2015) The Code for nurses and midwives: **www.nmc.org. uk/globalassets/sitedocuments/nmc-publications/nmc-code.pdf**,

This document clearly sets out the expected behaviours and actions that guide your practice as a developing professional nurse.

10. Royal College of Nursing (2014) *Defining Nursing*. London: Royal College of Nursing: **www. rcn.org.uk/about-us/our-history**

Chapter 2

Introduction to research, resources and academic practices

Stephen A. Bowman, Pamela Thomas, Adebisi Adelaja and Marian Brown

NMC Standards of Proficiency for Registered Nurses

Platform 1: Being an accountable professional

Registered nurses act in the best interests of people, putting them first and providing nursing care that is person-centred, safe and compassionate. They act professionally at all times and use their knowledge and experience to make evidence-based decisions about care. They communicate effectively, are role models for others, and are accountable for their actions. Registered nurses continually reflect on their practice and keep abreast of new and emerging developments in nursing, health and care.

At the point of registration, the registered nurse will be able to:

1.7   demonstrate an understanding of research methods, ethics and governance in order to critically analyse, safely use, share and apply research findings to promote and inform best nursing practice;

1.8   demonstrate the knowledge, skills and ability to think critically when applying evidence and drawing on experience to make evidence informed decisions in all situations.

Platform 5: Leading and managing nursing care and working in teams

Registered nurses provide leadership by acting as a role model for best practice in the delivery of nursing care. They are responsible for managing nursing care and are accountable for the appropriate delegation and supervision of care provided by others in the team, including lay carers. They play an active and equal role in the interdisciplinary team, collaborating and communicating effectively with a range of colleagues.

At the point of registration, the registered nurse will be able to:

5.11   effectively and responsibly use a range of digital technologies to access, input, share and apply information and data within teams and between agencies.

Chapter aims

....

After reading this chapter, you will be able to:

- undertake research using the processes, resources and support available through your library service;
- have the confidence to approach research and academic writing during your first year of study;
- understand and apply academic practices to prepare you for your course of study.

Introduction

University research is a constantly changing field. In this rapidly evolving environment this chapter will give you the information that you need to succeed. Over the last 20 years, the way that we research, the tools that we use and the resources that are available have changed fundamentally.

But don't panic! In this chapter we will discuss the research process (how you go about deciding on your approach to the subject), the use of the library facilities that will be available to you at most universities, the variety of resources to use for your assignments, the research tools that are available, and the academic practices that you will develop in order to write clearly and accurately for your lecturers.

The chapter begins with an outline of the publishing changes that are still taking place in the academic environment, specifically the move away from 'traditional' publishing practices to an 'open access' environment, and the impact of this on your research. It then moves on to discuss the higher education environment in which you will be working while on your course. The third section will examine the research tools that are available, including libraries, catalogues, discovery services and databases. The following section examines the resources themselves – monographs, journals, websites and online reading lists – that you will find in the majority of higher education institutions.

The chapter continues with an introduction to the academic practices that you will need and includes how to plan your first essay, how to brainstorm, critical thinking and analysis.

Research and resources

Publishing

Had you been entering your course of study in the last century you would have been faced with rooms full of printed journals (and printed indexes) that would need to be physically trawled over for the information that you would need to inform your writing. Over the last 30 years or so, the way in which journals are published and the ways in which they can be interrogated have changed fundamentally, and continue to do so. This has been driven in the most part by the technological changes that have impacted on all aspects of our lives. Most journals, and many monographs (books) are now available electronically, which makes the discovery of the information that you need far easier than in the past.

The other main driver for change in the publishing industry has been the move to 'open access' (OA) publishing. This move has been driven by the needs of researchers across the world for more rapid access to information as soon as it is discovered, rather than when it finally becomes published.

The concept summary below will introduce you to one of the main drivers changing the way that you can access academic research at university.

Concept summary

What is open access?

Open access is about making the products of research freely accessible to all. It allows research to be disseminated quickly and widely, the research process to operate more efficiently, and increased use and understanding of research by business, government, charities and the wider public.

Green and gold routes to open access

There are two complementary mechanisms for achieving open access to research.

The first mechanism is for authors to publish in open-access journals that do not receive income through reader subscriptions.

The second is for authors to deposit their refereed journal article in an open electronic archive. These two mechanisms are often called the 'gold' and 'green' routes to open access:

- **Gold** This means publishing in a way that allows immediate access to everyone electronically and free of charge. Publishers can recoup their costs through a number of mechanisms, including through payments from authors called article processing charges (APCs), or through advertising, donations or other subsidies.
- **Green** This means depositing the final peer-reviewed research output in an electronic archive called a repository. Repositories can be run by the researcher's institution, but shared or subject repositories are also commonly used. Access to the research output can be granted either immediately or after an agreed embargo period.

(HEFCE, 2017)

We will discuss more about the OA changes in the next section on the higher education landscape.

Higher education

This section will introduce you to the world of academia in which you will be working while you study.

The way that universities operate and are perceived has also changed over the past 30 years. In the past, they were seen as purveyors of self-improvement and self-development; more recently (and especially since the introduction of student fees), they are seen as routes to employment. In the past, universities often had a particular focus on either research (the Russell Group) or on teaching (the post-1992 universities). In this more competitive age, many universities are moving towards a more 'applied' approach to each of these areas.

One of the main determinants for a university's prestige and perception is the Research Excellence Framework (REF). This is an exercise run every seven years that examines the research outputs of an institution to gauge the impact of that institution's research on the wider world. The REF is co-ordinated by the four UK higher education funding bodies (www.rcuk.ac.uk/), which have introduced an open-access requirement in the next Research Excellence Framework. The outcome of this move has been that all research that is produced by UK universities that they wish to be considered for the next REF has to be published in an open access format. You can read more about this here: www.rcuk.ac.uk/documents/documents/rcukopenaccesspolicy-pdf/

With the two drivers of the changing publishing landscape and the championing of OA by the UK Research Councils, this has had a fundamental effect on the types of research materials that can be accessed by you on your course.

The next section will begin to look at the research environment and tools that you will come across while you are in your first year of study.

University research

You are a researcher! In your working day, you are researching all of the time, finding information about patients, conditions, interventions and outcomes. Within your university studies you will also be expected to undertake independent study and research as part of your course – indeed, the main focus of your course will be on independent study. The primary location for this independent study and research will be the university library. This section will introduce you to the generic library environment that you will find available in most universities.

Case study: Constance

Constance has just started her course in Occupational Health Nursing and is asked to find materials for her first assignment on Risk Assessments in the Workplace. She has some materials listed in her module guide and knows that most of her study will be self-directed. She heads for the library, but cannot find any of the journals that she needs on the shelves. In desperation, she turns to the library staff, who explain that most of the journal materials are now provided electronically and that this is done through the library Discovery Service. After some instruction, Constance is able to locate the materials that she needs for her assignment.

In the above case study, we can see that Constance may need the assistance of specialists within the library service at her university to help her locate the materials that she needs and hone the skills that she requires to become an independent learner as she progresses through her course.

University libraries

This section will introduce you to the academic library environment where most of your research and independent study will take place.

Libraries have been at the heart of universities and their work since they were first established. The University of Bologna, Italy, was founded in 1088 and is the oldest in Europe (www.guinnessworldrecords.com/world-records/oldest-university). University libraries have always sought to collect and maintain the widest selection of materials to support students in their studies. University libraries today still have the same mission. Unlike public libraries, which contain general reading materials that satisfy the needs of a wide range of the population, university libraries generally only hold those materials that support the programmes run by that institution. Therefore, you will find that when you are studying nursing in the university environment, there will be collections of materials that are specifically intended for the courses that you are studying. The technological advances mentioned earlier in this chapter have also had a huge impact on the 'shape' of academic libraries over the last 30 years. You will find that although virtually all academic libraries have collections of printed books and journals on the shelves, the vast majority of the information they contain is now available online. Therefore, the majority of the research that you carry out while at university will be accessed electronically. There are major benefits for you in this shift: first, searching for materials from a computer terminal (or from your own device) is far quicker and easier than reading through printed indexes and printed journals; second, online materials are always there and someone cannot remove that particular journal or book from its location, thus preventing you from finding the information that you need; third, you can generally access all the information you need either on or off campus with your university details. The resources that are available to you through your university library can generally be accessed via three routes.

The library catalogue

Academic library catalogues are available in many forms, but their functions are generally the same. The catalogue gives you access to the materials held by the library. Virtually all of the library catalogues that you will come across are now online. Some specialised collections may still offer access through a card-catalogue system, but these are very rare. Library catalogues will generally allow you to search for the materials that you need by subject, author, title or keyword.

A typical search box for an academic library catalogue allows you simply to type in the subjects or keywords that you want to find, and the catalogue then gives you the results. Most library catalogues will let you search the physical holdings of the library – hence, the printed books on the shelves and other physical materials such as CDs and DVDs, as well as the titles of any journals that the library holds in print.

Virtually all university library collections are arranged by a classification scheme. The most popular scheme in the UK is Dewey Decimal Classification, or DDC. The Dewey system allocates a number to every subject in the collection, so that all the materials on a given subject are likely to be in the same position within the library. For example:

'Medicine' in DDC can be found at 610 and is divided into the following categories:

- 610 Medicine and health
- 611 Human anatomy, cytology and histology
- 612 Human physiology
- 613 Personal health and safety
- 614 Incidence and prevention of disease
- 615 Pharmacology and therapeutics
- 616 Diseases
- 617 Surgery and related medical specialities
- 618 Gynaecology, obstetrics, paediatrics and geriatrics

(www.oclc.org/content/dam/oclc/dewey/DDC%2023_Summaries.pdf)

'Nursing' falls within this system at 610.73, so if you can find one book on nursing in your library catalogue, you can find them all on the shelf.

Many academic libraries now offer an extension to this online functionality in the form of a Discovery Service.

The Discovery Service

Web-scale discovery services — tools that search seamlessly across a wide range of local and remote content and provide relevance-ranked results — have the ambitious goal of providing a single point of entry into a library's collections . . . . Ideally all possible online content providers are indexed, as well as the library's local holdings.

(Breeding, 2014)

These Discovery Services are now widely available in most academic libraries. Rather than just giving access to the physical holdings of the library, the Discovery Service provides access to a vast range of resources to which the institution subscribes. These may include journals, monographs, databases, conference papers, dissertations, news articles, websites, trade publications and reviews. The third type of resource is the database, described in the following section.

Databases

Databases are collections of materials arranged around a certain subject. The larger databases will contain all of the academically produced materials in a chosen subject area. For nursing, the main database is the 'Cumulative Index of Nursing and Allied Health Literature', or CINAHL.

CINAHL is the definitive research tool for nursing and allied health professionals. The content of this database includes the following.

- Full text for more than 1,300 journals.
- Indexing for nearly 5,500 journals.
- Searchable cited references for more than 1,500 journals.
- Full text dating back to 1937.
- More than 5.8 million records.

(www.ebscohost.com/nursing/products/cinahl-databases/cinahl-complete)

Your university library will often have access to dozens of these subject-based databases, many of which will be searchable through the library's Discovery Service. Please be aware, however, that you will always find articles and other materials on a database search that you cannot access through your library system. This is because the databases list all the materials that are available, but your university may only subscribe to a selection of these.

Catalogue/Discovery Service/database tricks and tips

Computers are stupid

Although searching online materials can be very fast and can locate a vast range of resources to support your studies, machines are not human beings – they cannot (at the moment!) 'think'. If you type a word into a search box, the computer will just search for that word, not what that word may mean to you or me. For example:

I need to find materials on wellbeing. If I type the word 'wellbeing' into the computer, it will search for that word only; it will not search for 'well being' or 'well-being' – in the same way. If I make a mistake and search for 'intervntions', the computer will only find materials with that misspelling.

For this reason, always think about the 'aboutness' of the search words that you use. If you are searching for materials about young people, you may have to search for 'young people' or 'children' or 'toddlers' or 'infants' in order to find all the materials that are 'about' this subject.

There are also a number of features that are available across many online search systems that enable you to influence the results of the search – for example:

Truncation

You can often truncate a word to just a stem by using an asterisk – for example, nurs* in most systems will search for nurse, nurses, nursing, etc. You might use this if your original search term did not result in enough items located.

Wild cards

You can use a wildcard (often either # or ?) to replace any character – for example, wom#n will find woman or women. You may need to use this as many databases are compiled in the United States, with US spelling conventions.

Quotation marks

If you need to search for a phrase or a person's name, use quotation marks – for example, John Edwards (because computers are stupid) will just search for the word John and the word Edwards. However, if you put your search term in quotation marks – e.g. 'John Edwards' – the computer will know to search for those two words next to each other.

Activity 2.1 now asks you to put some of this information into practice.

Activity 2.1   Evidence-based practice and research

Use your Discovery Service/library catalogue to find materials. Go to your university library's catalogue page, where you will generally find a link to the Discovery Service that looks something like Figure 2.1 below.

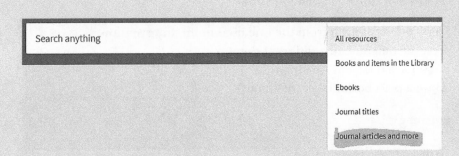

Figure 2.1   Example of a university library Discovery Service

This example comes from the University of Sussex library website and can be accessed at: https://sussex-primo.hosted.exlibrisgroup.com/

Search for a term or phrase that interests you. Remember that you can use truncation, wildcards and quotation marks with most search services to refine the results that you obtain.

As this answer is based on your particular institution, there is no outline answer at the end of the chapter.

Having practised using the catalogue in the library, we now look at a tool called PICO.

PICO

One of the main tools that you can use to examine a question and find the keywords that you need is called PICO. It is typically used in evidence-based practice to help you formulate and research your clinical question. You have an idea of what you want to find out, but realise you are unable to work out how to phrase it into a clinical question that can be answered. This is where PICO can help.

P: patient/population/problem

- Think about who you are looking at or what is the problem you are trying to solve.
- Is there a certain age group you would be looking at – elderly or perhaps children?
- Do your patients have a certain illness or disorder?
- Is your focus on people from a particular ethnicity or gender?

I: intervention

- Consider what is going to happen to your patient.
- Measure the effect of a particular drug.
- Examine the results of taking part in a specific therapy.
- Another form of treatment.

C: comparison (there is not always one)

- Try a different drug from the one used in the Intervention.
- Test the outcome of a different therapy.
- Observe a different treatment.
- Have a placebo (a 'fake' treatment).

O: outcome

- What do you hope to measure?
- Drug A improves the ailment better than drug B.
- Treatment A has a positive impact in comparison to treatment B.
- Treatment C and the placebo had the same outcome.

Once you have narrowed down your clinical question into PICO, the next step is to think of all the ways your concepts can be described. For example, there are many different ways of describing the 'elderly'. They can also be referred to as 'older adult', 'elder', 'geriatric', etc. The section above on 'Catalogue/Discovery Service/database tricks and tips' will explain why this is so important when you are conducting a search on the journal databases.

The next section will look at the various materials that are available through these tools and how they can support your studies.

Resources

Books (monographs)

For centuries, libraries have been constructed around the book. Books (either in print or online form) are still an important part of the information that you will need to access for your studies. Books provide an excellent source if you are looking for the background or development of a particular subject. If you are looking at the history of nursing, the history of the NHS, the history of diseases or the development of the nursing profession, then books should be your first choice.

Books in general deal with a broad subject area. They generally take one to two years to be published, so should not be used for current research. If you are looking for up-to-date information, statistics, etc., you should look to the journals.

An excellent book which covers the subjects in this chapter can be linked to at: (https://uk.sagepub.com/en-gb/eur/understanding-research-for-nursing-students/book245597)

Journals (periodicals)

Academic journals (or periodicals) are subject-based publications that are issued on a frequent basis, so a journal may be published on a monthly, quarterly or biannual basis.

This frequency of publication, along with the specific subject nature of most journals, makes them the ideal choice if you wish to capture up-to-date information, statistics and research in your chosen field. Each issue of a journal will have individual articles written by experts in that subject. You are far more likely to find a range of journal articles in a very specific subject than you are to find a monograph on that subject. In order to search the institution's journals, head for the Discovery Service or the databases.

An excellent journal which covers the subjects in this chapter can be linked to at: http://0-journals.sagepub.com.lispac.lsbu.ac.uk/home/njna

Online reading lists

Many universities now offer online reading lists as part of their service. These online reading lists are generally compiled by your lecturers and give you instant access to many of the core resources for your course or module. Unlike the printed reading lists of old, these will offer you links to a range of online materials such as e-books, e-journals, websites, and more. These lists can change across the academic year, so it is always a good idea to go back to your list periodically to check if new materials have been added by your lecturer.

Websites

Most of the materials that you will need for your research while at university will be available through the library service and your online reading lists. However, if you are looking for materials outside the academic realm, such as reports by central or local government, policies and procedures, materials from trusts and non-governmental organisations (NGOs), then you may have to look on the open Web. Bear in mind at all times that the internet is an 'open' space. Anyone can upload materials to the Web, and you must be vigilant about the authority of any materials that may be found there. If in doubt about Web-based materials, approach your library service for advice.

e-books and journals

As we mentioned earlier in this chapter, many journals and books are now available in electronic formats. These are likely to be searchable through each of the tools above (Catalogues, Discovery Service, Databases). The main point to note is that these are 'just' electronic versions of the original materials. An e-book is just a copy of a printed book that is available online; e-books have the same drawbacks as printed books in that they take a considerable time to be published, and they are fixed in time at that point. As previously noted, the positive points about e-materials are that they are available 24/7, and that they are easily searchable online. A further source of information, which lies outside the academic publishing arena, are theses.

Audio-visual materials

All university libraries will also contain collections of audio-visual materials that you can access. These may be in the form of DVDs that you can borrow or as online resources that are non-text based. These may include resources on anatomy and physiology, physical examination techniques and other subjects presented visually.

Theses

A thesis is an extended essay or dissertation involving personal research, written by a candidate for a university degree. In the UK, all doctoral theses can be accessed through the British Library's EThOS service (http://ethos.bl.uk/Home.do). If you are researching a particular subject area and wish to discover whether research has already been undertaken in this area, you can search EThOS by subject or keyword.

The majority of theses available through EThOS are instantly (and freely) downloadable, either directly through EThOS or from the awarding university.

Activity 2.2   Evidence-based practice and research

Find a thesis by one of your lecturers on EThOS. Go to the EThOS website: http://ethos.bl.uk/Home.do. Enter your lecturer's name in the search box and see what results you obtain. (NB: Your lecturer would need to have been awarded a doctorate for their thesis to be available through the EThOS service.)

As this answer is based on your own observation, there is no outline answer at the end of the chapter.

We now move on to look at the academic skills that you will need to produce assignments and reports that will shine.

Academic literacy practices

You are now embarking upon a journey of academic and professional discovery. This section of the chapter will introduce you to the fundamentals of the academic essay writing process, critical thinking and the analytical processes that you will learn and develop. As a pre-registration nursing student, learning how to study is important and you must to be able to approach all your assessments in a strategic and systematic way to become a successful and independent nursing practitioner with good written and oral communication skills (Northedge, 2005; Whitehead, 2002).

Getting to grips with academic writing

Writing is a process that takes time to develop and master. As an undergraduate pre-registration nursing student, you will be introduced to many different academic writing styles. These may consist of a traditional academic essay, a reflective account, a care plan, a narrative recount, a discharge plan, a care critique, a discharge summary or a case study (Gimenez, 2008). One form of assessment that you will be asked to do is to write the traditional academic essay. Here, we will take you through the process of how to plan your first academic essay.

What is an academic essay?

An essay is a piece of writing on a particular topic and is structured in paragraphs. Each paragraph forms the basis of the essay and consists of three main parts – an introductory paragraph, body paragraph and a concluding paragraph.

- An introduction sets the scene and introduces the topic of the essay. It also contains an important sentence that clearly states the main idea of the essay. This is called the thesis statement.
- The main body is made up of several paragraphs; each paragraph explains and develops one part of the essay topic.
- The conclusion is the final paragraph and summarises the main body of the essay.

In higher education, an essay is a very common form of assessment and it allows you, as the writer, to demonstrate your knowledge and skill on a particular topic within your discipline. You will also be able to show your lecturer that you can voice your opinion on a specific topic and articulate it through your essay.

The essay writing process

When you begin your first writing assignment, it is very easy to become overwhelmed by the writing process, especially if you have never written academically. Be prepared to allocate enough time to brainstorm the topic, develop a plan, research the topic and, most importantly, set aside the time to write. Once you have been given the assignment task, you should start to think about how to break the task down so that you understand all the component parts of the essay in order to fully understand the requirements. The beginning of an essay is the most important stage in the writing process, as having a clear direction and focus will allow you to investigate the topic through your research and begin your first draft of the essay. Is it important to note that a draft is a rough document that is not smooth or polished in any way, so you don't have to worry about it looking perfect at this stage. Within the essay writing process, the following steps – read and interpret the assignment task, brainstorm the essay topic and make a preliminary plan – will set you up well and are the groundwork for producing any writing task now and in the future.

Read, interpret and understand the assignment question

The first step, and the most important part of the essay planning process, is to interpret the essay title so that you are clear about what is being asked of you, so you can answer the question set in a structured way: an introduction, a main body and a conclusion as outlined above in 'What is an academic essay?'

Essay titles usually contain key words, often called 'instruction words' as they tell you what you need to do in the essay. An instruction word – for example, *discuss, analyse, explain, describe, outline, define* – will guide your approach to the task and show you exactly what you need to do. Be sure that you note and understand these key words, because if you misinterpret or do not clearly understand their meaning, you could end up writing a well-prosed essay and unfortunately not answer the question correctly (Gillet, 2018).

Activity 2.3 now asks you to consider what an essay title is really asking.

Activity 2.3   Critical thinking

Match the instruction word found in the assignment task with the definition that best describes what the lecturer wants you to do.

Instruction word	Definition
Examine	Give the main features or the general principles of the subject.
Evaluate	Examine and analyse all sides of the issue. Reach a conclusion.
Discuss	Break it down into its components/elements.
Analyse	Make plain and interpret. Simplify the material to present. Give reasons for important features and developments. Attempt to analyse causes.
Assess	Weighing up the relative strengths and weaknesses; points for and against; advantages or disadvantages.
Explain	Make a reasoned judgement about the value or legitimacy of a particular argument, concept or theory.

An outline answer is provided at the end of the chapter.

From understanding the essay question, we now turn to how to gather the information needed to write the essay.

Brainstorming for your essay

Brainstorming is a way of generating ideas, theories, concepts and solutions to activate knowledge about a particular topic (Businessballs.com, 2017). It is a way for you to write down any thoughts or reflections you may have in your research and writing. At this stage you are noting down anything you already know about the topic. Do you already have evidence you can use? If so, which medium? Here is a good time to question the question itself as you will be able to brainstorm all the possibilities, the scope and any limitations of the topic/question. It is important to keep the title close to hand and remain focused when you begin to write your first draft.

Activity 2.4 Decision-making, reflection, critical thinking

Consider the following scenario.

Naomi has now completed her first few weeks at university and has settled in well. She has enjoyed attending her lectures, seminars and has been assigned a personal tutor. At a meeting with her personal tutor, they discuss putting together an outline of her assessments so she can have an overview of all the different types of assessments she will need to complete, as well as when they are due for submission. At home, Naomi is going through each of her module guides and noticed that she has to write a 1,500 word essay, which is due much sooner than she first envisaged, on 'Is nursing still seen as a caring profession? Discuss.'

What steps you would recommend to Naomi on how to begin her essay?

A possible answer is provided at the end of the chapter.

When working on an assignment, remember to print out your work at regular intervals. Examining your work on paper allows you to focus on the content away from the glare and distraction of a computer screen. Lastly, make sure you have allocated enough time to draft and redraft your work.

Critical thinking

Whether undertaking an essay, care plan or other written coursework, or when dealing with clients, you are expected to keep an open mind before making a decision. We will now look at another key skill required to become a successful nursing professional, a practice used for applying practical and theoretical knowledge known as critical thinking. The critical thinking process involves questioning all forms of spoken and written information that you come across.

The key to becoming a successful critical thinker is in developing a critical outlook ('mindset'), *inside* and *outside* of the classroom (McKendry, 2016).

Being critical for academic study

As stated earlier, the ability to be critical is essential for academic study. Subsequently, in order to fulfil assessment criteria you will need to demonstrate that you are critically aware in a *purposeful* way. Critiquing can be challenging, especially if you may not have done it before. Ultimately, your lecturers are looking for proof that you have understood how to *analyse* (break up into parts and investigate in detail), *evaluate* (assess the value of information) and *synthesise* your ideas (combine research from a variety of sources) (Giminez, 2007). Always remember that there is often more than one answer to an issue or problem. However, you should have come to a decision after *careful consideration* of the evidence.

Critical questions to ask and answer

The following is a series of open-ended questions that highlight the critical thinking process, questions that can be applied to any situation (in health and social care, situations that occur in practice are often described as *incidents* or *scenarios*).

- Question 1: Explaining and exploring – what happened?
- Question 2: Analysing and challenging – how did it happen? why did it happen? what are the valuable and significant factors? what could have been different?
- Question 3: Examining and reflection – what has been learnt? what should you do next?

(adapted from Giminez, 2007)

Activity 2.5   Reflection

Think of an incident you have dealt with in a work situation. Reflect on the situation by addressing the critical questions above.

As this activity is based on your own observations, there is no outline answer at the end of the chapter.

Critical reading

Developing a critical approach to reading involves reading *purposely* with your question in mind. You are reading effectively when you understand *how* to read the text – for example, skimming, sampling or in detail – and *why* are you reading the text.

Strategy for critical reading (www.nhs.uk/news/)

When critiquing research, always think about the following questions:

- Where did the story come from?
- What kind of research was this?
- What did the research involve?
- What were the basic results?
- How did the researcher (or researchers) explain the results?

Overall, you are making a judgement as to the *validity* (is it accurate?), *credibility* (is it believable?), *reliability* (can it be reproduced?) and *rigour* (is it exact/consistent?) of information (Ellis, 2016b).

Scenario

Your lecturer has written an article about the effectiveness of natural remedies on cancer survival rates. The same lecturer has been in the nursing profession for 25 years. Should you question what they have written? The answer is 'yes!' Even though your lecturer has been in the profession for a number of years, they would still expect you to treat their article exactly the same as any other research. Therefore, whatever the source, it is important to be critical; this involves looking for strengths, weaknesses, gaps in the research and limitations of the study.

Descriptive v. critical writing

Students who do not provide enough evidence of critical thinking often receive the following feedback from their lecturers about their written work: 'too descriptive'; 'lacks critical analysis'.

Academic projects always require a level of descriptive information to inform the reader about the task. One of the reasons that students are told their work is too descriptive is that they have included details that may be interesting, but are *irrelevant* for the assignment.

It should be acknowledged that, on occasion, lecturers instruct students that their work is too descriptive, but forget to provide further clarification of how to improve the critical aspects of the writing (Wingate, 2011).

Look at the following example taken from case notes. The paragraph was focused around the assessment of a patient (the unnecessary details are in italic).

'The family were present throughout the assessment to ensure that guidelines were correctly enforced. . . . *Medication was administered at 4pm, 6pm and 10pm that day.*

Use of one of the following phrases would have improved the paragraph and made it more critical – for example:

As a consequence . . . As a result . . .

The implication being that . . .

Developing a critical mindset takes time

Ellis (2016a, p82) describes the importance of *personal as well as professional experience* in the nursing profession. The importance of a 'sixth sense' or a 'gut' feeling that we may have in our personal or professional lives, which is often based on situations we have encountered, may come in useful, but should not be relied upon to make a judgement.

Our perception of a situation may be *subjective* (for example, our individual experience of pain) or *objective* (evidence based). Consequently, being critical involves reflecting on subjective and objective experiences so that you make *reasoned* and *informed* decisions.

Chapter summary

This chapter has introduced you to the environment in which you will be studying at university. It has shown you examples of the ways in which you can access the materials that you need to find to support your studies, and the various kinds of materials that you will come across while researching. The chapter concluded with an overview of the academic practices and skills that you will need in order to produce well-researched and written coursework. The following chapters will introduce you to the range of professional skills necessary for a successful first year as a nursing student.

Activities: Brief outline answers

Activity 2.3   Critical thinking (p46)

Defining key words in essay titles

Instruction word	Definition
Examine	Present the situation in depth.
Evaluate	Make a reasoned judgement about the value or legitimacy of a particular argument, concept or theory.
Discuss	Examine and analyse all sides of the issue. Reach a conclusion.
Analyse	Break it down into its components/elements.
Assess	Weighing up the relative strengths and weaknesses; points for and against; advantages or disadvantages.
Explain	Make plain and interpret. Simplify the material to present. Give reasons for important features and developments. Attempt to analyse causes.

Activity 2.4   Decision-making, reflection, critical thinking (p00)

What steps you would recommend to Naomi on how to begin her essay?

The steps outlined below have been broken down into smaller steps. Plan each step along the way, setting yourself deadlines for completion of each task and trying to keep to the deadline.

Cottrell (1999) outlines a number of key steps of the essay writing process.

1. Receive the topic/question.

2. Interpret the assignment task or question.

3. Brainstorm the essay topic/subject area and make a preliminary plan.

4. Source your reading material; make notes and record bibliographic information.

5. Draft your first piece of writing.

6. Review, rewrite and review your draft.

7. Compile your reference list.

8. Proofread and finalise for submission.

In Step 2, a very important part of the initial writing process is to interpret the question and ask questions of the question before moving on to Step 3. It is not uncommon to incorporate both Steps 2 and 3 together; however, try to attempt Step 2 to gain a good, clear interpretation of the essay title or task before proceeding.

What may be recommended to Naomi on how to begin her essay would be to invest quality time to break down and analyse the essay title, 'Is nursing still seen as a caring profession? Discuss.' Below is an outline of how to interpret her essay writing assignment as set out by Gillet (2018).

1. **Subject matter or topic** What, in the most general terms, is the question about?	Nursing.
2. **Aspect or focus** This is the angle or point of view on the subject matter. What aspect of the subject matter is the question about?	Still a caring profession?
3. **Instruction or comment** The instruction word tells you exactly what to do.	Discuss.
4. **Restriction or expansion of the subject matter** This is the detailed limitation of the topic. What, in specific terms, is the question about?	Expansion: still, up to and including the present time.
5. **Viewpoint** This refers to the requirement, in the question, that the writer writes from the point of view dictated by the setter of the question.	Yes, there is a viewpoint. What is your view of the nursing profession? Is it still caring – yes/no or indifferent? You are the one to decide this and examine, analyse and reach a conclusion on the subject matter.

Further reading

Cottrell, S (2017) *Critical Thinking Skills: Effective Analysis, Argument and Reflection* (3rd edn).
Basingstoke: Palgrave Macmillan.

An accessible guide to the critical thinking process for all levels of study.

Crème, P and Lea, MR (1997) *Writing at University: A Guide for Students.* Maidenhead: McGraw-Hill/ Open University Press.

An insightful book that outlines traditional essays and other forms of university writing.

McMillian, K and Weyes, J (2006) *The Smarter Student: Study Skills and Strategies for Success at University.* Harlow: Pearson Education.

A handy book of tips and techniques to develop essential study skills and strategies.

Payne, E and Whittaker, L (2006) *Developing Essential Study Skills* (2nd edn). Harlow: Pearson Education.

A comprehensive study skills book with a pragmatic approach for pre-university students from any discipline.

Useful websites

www.nhs.uk/news/

Section of the NHS website that examines clinical evidence behind the headlines. Each category – for example, food and diet, medication – provides clear explanation of how and why the research was carried out. A link to the original journal article that each headline is based on is also provided.

www.uefap.net/

Gillet, A (2018) *Using English for Academic Purposes for Students in Higher Education.* This website is a non-discipline specific website with great examples of how writing in the university setting is a necessary academic practice to be developed.

www.open.ac.uk/goodstudyguide

Northedge, A (2005) *The Good Study Guide* (2nd edn). Milton Keynes: Open University Press.

A companion guide to the book with excellent resources for the challenges of studying in higher education where computers and the internet are commonplace.

Chapter 3 Communication in nursing

Calvin Moorley, Xabi Cathala and
Nova Corcoran

NMC Standards of Proficiency for Registered Nurses

Platform 1: Being an accountable professional

Registered nurses act in the best interests of people, putting them first and providing nursing care that is person-centred, safe and compassionate. They act professionally at all times and use their knowledge and experience to make evidence-based decisions about care. They communicate effectively, are role models for others and are accountable for their actions. Registered nurses continually reflect on their practice and keep abreast of new emerging developments in nursing, health and care.

At the point of registration, the registered nurse will be able to:

1.11 Communicate effectively using a range of skills and strategies with colleagues and people at all stages of life and with a range of mental, physical, cognitive and behavioural health challenges.

Platform 2: Promoting health and preventing ill health

Registered nurses play a key role in improving and maintaining the mental, physical and behavioural health and well-being of people, families, communities and populations. They support and enable people at all stages of life and in all care settings to make informed choices about how to manage health challenges in order to maximise their quality of life and improve health outcomes. They are actively involved in the prevention of and protection against disease and ill health and engage in public health, community development and global health agendas, and in the reduction of health inequalities.

2.9 Use appropriate communication skills and strength-based approaches to support and enable people to make informed choices about their care to manage health challenges in order to have satisfying and fulfilling lives within the limitations caused by reduced capability, ill health and disability.

(Continued)

(Continued)

Platform 4: Providing and evaluating care

Registered nurses take the lead in providing evidence-based, compassionate and safe nursing interventions. They ensure that care they provide and delegate is person-centred and of a consistently high standard. They support people of all ages in a range of care settings. They work in partnership with people, families and carers to evaluate whether care is effective, and the goals of care have been met in line with their wishes, preferences and desired outcomes.

4.3 Demonstrate the knowledge, communication and relationship management skills required to provide people, families and carers with accurate information that meets their needs before, during and after a range of interventions.

Chapter aims

After reading this chapter, you will be able to:

* identify the different modes of communication;
* understand the various ways to communicate effectively with patients, their families and carers from diverse population groups;
* outline how to deliver patient-targeted health promotion through the appropriate use and delivery of patient information and education;
* describe ways to use online communication, including social media for professional nursing purposes.

Introduction

Case study: Ms Jones

Ms Jones is a 57-year-old patient who has had a right hip replacement and been transferred to your ward for ongoing rehabilitation from another area of the hospital. She has a husband and three children – two sons and a daughter. On transfer, she tells you that she is deaf in her right ear, but that she has already texted her family using her mobile phone and updated her social media status so that all her friends know where to come and visit her.

This case study is not unusual in the nursing profession and most student nurses would have had some experience of having to communicate with a patient, their carer and/or family. This chapter has started with the above case study to help illustrate how, as a student nurse, you will have to demonstrate effective communication in a variety of ways.

This chapter begins with looking at the different ways of communicating and then gets you to reflect on your communication skills. After this, you will be introduced to the different types of communication followed by how to communicate with different groups effectively, and sending and receiving messages. You will also learn about barriers to communication, communication channels and how to communicate with patients using mass media. The chapter ends on how to communicate health messages to different cultural groups and effectively use technology to communicate professionally, including the use of social media.

Activity 3.1 is designed to help you think how you will begin to communicate.

Activity 3.1   Critical thinking

In this activity, think about how we communicate with people. Make a list of the different ways in which you may need to communicate from the case study above.

An outline answer is provided at the end of the chapter.

The activity above was designed to help you think of the various ways you can communicate. This chapter is written and designed to help you develop your communication skills for nursing practice. *Communication is a transactional process . . . and vital in the achievement of healthy individuals* (Corcoran, 2013, p5). It involves the exchange of information and is both expert generated (the nurse) and user generated (the patient) (Thackeray and Neiger, 2009). We all have communication skills and this may be at an elementary, intermediate or advanced level, and may be as a result of your experience in working with people and caring for patients. As a student, you will need to develop your communication skills and be able to demonstrate this development, and your mentors will make comments and provide support to help you improve your communication skills. This chapter focuses on three main types of communication skills: verbal, written and non-verbal using body language, including facial expressions.

Activity 3.2 is designed to help you assess your communication skills.

Activity 3.2   Reflection

Part 1 Rating your communication skills

Reflect on a situation in clinical practice where you have had to communicate before completing the exercise below.

Where 1 = poor skills and 5 = excellent, please rate yourself on the following:

Verbal communication: 1   2   3   4   5

Written communication: 1   2   3   4   5

Non verbal, including facial and body language communication: 1   2   3   4   5

Part 2 Identifying your strengths and areas for development

For each type of communication skill in Part 1, we would like you to make a list of what you do really well and what you can improve on. For example, in verbal communication, you may identify your strength as being able to speak clearly, and your area for development may be to make eye contact when speaking to others.

As this is a reflective exercise based on a self-assessment of your communication skills, no outline answer is provided.

Now that you have self-rated your communication skills and identified your strengths and areas for development, in the next section we focus on the various types of communication.

Types of communication

There are two main types of communication when relaying a message: verbal and non-verbal. Verbal communication involves the use of speech to transfer or communicate the message to the other person, and concerns the words, sentences and phrases used (Minardi and Riley, 1997). Non-verbal communication is concerned with any form of information transmission that does not involve speech, and includes eye contact, gestures, intonation, rhythm – i.e. speed – and factors such as the appearance of the sender (Corcoran, 2013).

Types of verbal communication

When you communicate with someone verbally, you can do so either directly or indirectly. In the case study introducing Ms Jones, you can communicate directly by addressing the patient – for example, you may say 'Welcome to the ward, Ms Jones, my name is Calvin and I will be your nurse today'. Here, you will be talking directly to the patient and she could respond directly to you. The communication may continue with you providing Ms Jones with a tour of the ward. There are other environments to which patients will be admitted, such as day surgery, or they may be in an outpatient area, in which case you will still need to introduce yourself and show the patient around as required. Activity 3.3 is designed to help you think about how you can use your communication skills when admitting a patient to the ward or clinical area.

Activity 3.3   Reflection

Make a list of what information you think you will need to communicate to a patient on admission. No outline answer is provided, but possible answers are discussed in the section below.

After completing the activity in this section, you should have a good idea of what information needs to be communicated to the patient on admission. In the next section, we discuss some of these areas and how to communicate effectively with different groups.

It is important that you acknowledge and understand that admission to hospital can be very worrying for a patient and their family and/or carers. The ward and the activities that take place can be overwhelming for the patient. The ward setting can be an unfamiliar area, as well as intimidating for the patient. Therefore, you will need to use your communication skills to help place the patient at ease and make them feel welcomed and as comfortable as possible.

You may want to use the SOLER communication model developed by Gerard Egan (1998) for non-verbal listening in communication. It is an acronym that stands for:

S   Sit *squarely* to the client/patient; a 5 o'clock position is better, which avoids the possibility of staring.

O   Try to maintain an *open* posture throughout. Avoid crossing your arms or legs, which can appear defensive.

L   *Lean* slightly in towards the client/patient.

E   Maintain *eye contact* with the client/patient, but ensure that you are not staring.

R   *Relax* – being relaxed can help to put the client/patient at ease.

Egan developed other guidance and tips for communication; you can read more about them in the Useful websites section at the end of the chapter.

Some of the information you will need to communicate to the patient on admission is as follows:

- Inform the patient of the layout of the ward, which will include where the sitting room is located, the location of the bathroom and the nurses' station.
- Show the patient where the nurse call bell is situated and demonstrate how to use it.
- You will also need to provide information on visiting times. This information may be in written form and you could read it together with the patient so that they are clear on the information.
- You will need to communicate hospital policies – e.g. no smoking, and also ward visiting times and how many visitors are allowed to visit at any one time.
- Very importantly, you will need to communicate information on meal times and whether family and visitors are allowed during this time. The patient may also have questions on bringing in their own food and heating provisions, such as using a microwave.
- Other information may include the use of mobile devices – e.g. smart phones and tablets, iPads – hospital Wi-Fi connection, hiring of television, important phone numbers and spiritual support services.

This interaction forms a direct communication. In your professional nursing experience, you will encounter many direct communications. Can you identify any other forms of direct communication you may encounter in your professional nursing career?

Types of non-verbal communication

Indirect communication is when you transmit a message to the individual using speech, but you use pauses and silences. These are vocal, but non-verbal in nature such as 'uh-huh' or 'mmm'. You do this when you do not want to indicate agreement or disagreement with the person. Sometimes, with indirect communication you may need to be firm but always polite.

Communicating effectively with different groups

It is important to understand that an individual's belief, experience of hospitals and illness and background can impact on how you communicate with them. Social variables such as ethnicity, culture or religion can impact on communication in numerous ways, including comprehension of information, beliefs around Western medicine, and different values and beliefs around health (Corcoran, 2013). It is also important to acknowledge cultural beliefs and values in the patient's explanations for their illness, as this may impact on how they respond to health promotion advice (Moorley et al., 2016). This suggests that patient communication may have to be adapted to be appropriate to diverse population groups, and that as a nurse you may have to adapt your communication style. For example, Brooke et al. (2017) suggest that understanding dementia, and the provision of care and support, are influenced by healthcare workers' culture. In some cultural groups, dementia is associated with negative spiritual forces such as black magic, voodoo or obeah.

Activity 3.4 asks you to explore how your own culture may influence the way in which you communicate with patients. It helps you to think of cultural diversity and being aware of your own and other people's culture.

Activity 3.4   Critical thinking

Make a list of the following:

1. How does your culture say you should address older or younger people?

2. How does your culture view mental health?

3. Make a list of how your cultural beliefs may impact on the way you communicate healthcare information.

Guidance is provided at the end of the chapter on how you may approach answering this activity.

Now that you have looked at how your own culture may impact on the care you provide, we will now look at how you communicate with patients, their families and carers.

As a nurse, you will have to communicate with patients, their families and carers. As we have seen so far in this chapter, communication can take different forms. You may also have to communicate to groups of patients or on a one-to-one basis. In this section, we look at one-to-one verbal communication. One-to-one, as its name suggests, is when you are communicating with only one other person.

The ability to communicate effectively with patients can help to build a trusting relationship and provide the appropriate care required. In the healthcare setting one-to-one communication can occur face-to-face or via a telephone or other type of media – e.g. FaceTime or Skype. It is usually when you have to give or gain information, which can be results or details about a procedure or explaining a disease process to a patient, or the patient may have questions which they need answering or clarifying. The way you communicate can alleviate the patient's fears and allow you to understand their concerns, or it can increase fears and anxiety. There are some areas you should consider when you are in a one-to-one communication situation.

One-to-one communication is a linear process and has the following components:

Sender: this is the person who is delivering the message.

Receiver: this is the person who receives the message.

Message: this is the information that is transmitted.

The way the message is delivered has two parts:

Encoding: this is the process of turning your thoughts into a communication (message), which is what the sender does.

Decoding: this is the process of turning the communication into a thought to make sense of what the sender is saying.

Sending and receiving messages accurately

It is important that when you are communicating, you send and receive accurate messages. In a busy hospital ward, you or the patient may unintentionally send the wrong message. Therefore, you need to choose words the receiver (the patient) will understand. This will depend on the social variables that we discussed earlier. Table 3.1 below provides some useful do's and don'ts that you may find helpful when engaging in one-to-one communication.

Communication do's	Communication don'ts
Use language and terms that the patient will understand.	Don't use language the patient will not be familiar with, such as nursing and medical jargon.
Make eye contact.	Don't look away from the patient when speaking.
Consider your physical position and aim to be at the same level as the patient.	Don't stand over the patient and speak to them.
Always use appropriate body language.	Don't use negative body language, such as folding arms, displaying boredom – e.g. tapping fingers or pen.
Always provide factual information.	Don't give your own opinions.
Ensure your audience understands what you are saying – e.g. seek clarification if necessary.	Don't assume that the patient has understood what you have said; you can confirm by asking the patient to paraphrase what you have said.
Assess if the patient needs an interpreter or a support device such as a hearing aid.	Don't assume your patient speaks and understands English or has full hearing.
Always maintain patient confidentiality.	Don't discuss conversations with third parties without the patient's consent.
Always be honest and truthful with a patient. It helps to build a trusting relationship. Always apply duty of candour when communicating with the patient.	Don't withhold or conceal information from the patient. The patient has the right to know everything that is related to their care and health.

Table 3.1 Communication do's and don'ts

Barriers to effective communication

Communication can also be influenced by external factors and you need to be aware of these. Hospitals are busy environments and the setting you are in may not lend itself to effective communication. You should be mindful of the level of noise and how this can impact on the conversation. Be aware of the environment and whether it allows for confidentiality and privacy for sensitive discussions. On a busy ward, you may have third-party interruptions, in which someone who is not part of your conversation interrupts you to ask a question – for example, another patient's relative asking you a 'quick' question. If you are using a telephone or another type of media apart from those stated above, you should check the line and network connections, and confirm you are speaking to the correct patient, asking them for their name, date of birth and address, or patient identification number.

Case study: Mr Tassi

Mr Tassi is a 68-year-old man of Ghanaian heritage. He has been admitted to your ward for a small bowel obstruction. Four years ago he was diagnosed with dementia (his wife believes there are non-medical causes for his dementia). He is very forgetful and does not sit for more than 30 minutes at a time.

Activity 3.5 asks you to use the case study about Mr Tassi to help you put your one-to-one communication skills into practice.

Activity 3.5   Team working

You have to explain to Mr Tassi that he will need to have surgery. Find a group of your peers and discuss how you will communicate this information to him. You may want to make a flow chart to organise your ideas.

As this is a group exercise, no outline answer is provided.

Now you will have worked as a team to address giving information to a patient and their family, explaining clinical conditions and listening to lay beliefs of health. In the next section we look at the different channels of communication.

Channels of communication

There are numerous and different ways, or channels, in which messages can be delivered to patients. Corcoran (2011) splits channels of communication into the three sections of interpersonal, organisations and community. Interpersonal is individual one-to-one communication, such as you discussing a behaviour change with a patient. You can also communicate through different organisations – i.e. the hospital, such as the flu vaccine messages you might see on television screens or websites in hospitals or at your university. You can also use community settings such as local community radio. Much of your work in a hospital setting will be interpersonal communication, which is when you work with patients and their families to give information about their health condition or information designed to improve their health in some way. This might be discussing how to take medication, reducing pressure injury risks by encouraging movement, or advice to help them manage their health when they leave the hospital, such as using an epi pen for diabetes or increasing their physical activity levels.

There are a number of things to consider when you are communicating with individuals. The main criticism by a number of authors is that the individualistic approach predominately focuses on the patient and not on the environment and social circumstances where they live. Health is created within the settings of where people live their everyday life (WHO, 1986), and thus attempts to improve patients' health will need to consider where they live. Individual health is influenced by social, physical and environmental contexts (Talbot and Verrinder, 2009), so one-to-one communication needs to acknowledge this. This includes knowing where to refer patients to for support with behaviour change – for example, a local leisure centre that offers women-only swimming sessions, a community centre that runs a weight-loss clinic or a pharmacist's that gives good stop-smoking support. Activity 3.6 asks you to look at using your knowledge of a local area to identify barriers and enablers for a healthy lifestyle.

Activity 3.6 Critical thinking

You are working with a patient who is overweight. You have advised them to continue to exercise when they are discharged from hospital and return home. Imagine that they live in a local area you are familiar with.

1. What things might be barriers or facilitators to continuing to exercise?

2. What resources are available in the local area that might help them to continue to exercise?

An outline answer is provided at the end of the chapter.

Having completed Activity 3.6, you will now have a better idea of how to communicate health promotion to a patient. As a nurse, you need to remember that communication may also occur between the patient and their friends and family, which will impact on the way they respond to your advice. This may be positive – for example, family members helping to support someone to reduce fat or sugar in their diet. Involving family members in interpersonal communication means that you will feel better equipped to support a patient.

Communicating patient education using mass media

The communication of information between nurses and patients is an important part of how nurses do their job (McCabe and Timmins, 2016). The provision of information, particularly complex information, can be supported by the use of mass media and may be better presented in this format (Corcoran, 2013). It may help patients to remember details or follow instructions that cannot be retained through a verbal conversation. It is not enough to use mass media by itself, however, and ideally you should talk the patient through the resource and explain why it will help them.

Commonly used resources in the broader field of health promotion and education include television, radio, electronic media such as the internet or smartphones, and print-based media such as leaflets or booklets. You may have access to different types of media that patients can take home with them – for example, DVDs – but commonly, leaflets and booklets are most frequently used. The internet and smart phones may have a range of resources that are useful for patients, but you should ensure that these are recommended by your place of work for use with patients – for example, apps to stop smoking or calculating alcohol units. One good source of patient support that may be overlooked are charity or voluntary organisations that have a wide range of patient resources available on the internet. The best way to get used to using different resources and seeing which ones you prefer are to have a look at the different resources that are available to help support patients and their families. Particularly good websites include Macmillan Cancer Support, British Heart Foundation, Age UK, Diabetes UK and The Samaritans (see Useful website links at the end of the chapter).

Adapting patient education to different cultural groups

Some population groups may require additional adaptations to the standard patient education and information that you might usually deliver. For example, for patients with a visual impairment you may need a non-written format or a larger font material. For those patients with specific learning disabilities, you may need resources that are easier to comprehend, such as those that use pictures and less text (see the next activity for an example). For better message design, health practitioners need to be able to identify influences on health behaviours (Huff et al., 2014). This means that as a nurse, you need to know what might influence the health of the patient in the broader context of who they are and where they live. A wide variety of health education resources are available, many of which have adaptations that might be useful for your patient group – for example, leaflets and booklets may be available in different languages or aimed at specific at-risk patient groups. In Activity 3.7, we ask you to look at a health promotion communication for people with learning disabilities.

Activity 3.7   Critical thinking

Look at the following resource for breast cancer patients, written for people with learning disabilities: https://assets.publishing.service.gov.uk/government/uploads/system/uploads/attachment_data/file/765594/Easy_guide_to_breast_screening.pdf

What things do you think are helpful in this resource for readers?

An outline answer is provided at the end of the chapter.

From Activity 3.7 you would have realised that when communicating health, the resource should be readable and suitable for the patient or patient group. You can work out how readable and suitable a leaflet or booklet is by applying a variety of 'tests' to a written resource. Readability is the level of accessibility of a written text that is often assumed by calculating the reading grade level of materials. You can also look at readability by ensuring that the resource tries to limit words that are two syllables or less – for example, 'pat-ient' is two syllables and 'hos-pi-tal' is three syllables. Suitability of a health education resource is an assessment of how appropriate a health resource (i.e. a leaflet) is for the target group in which it is intended – for example, attractiveness or cultural appropriateness. The Suitability Assessment of Materials (SAM) can be used to check the appropriateness of resources; a scoresheet for this is available at the Department of Health and Human Services (2018). Generally, if a patient finds something appealing or if a resource looks as if it is designed for someone like them, the more likely they are to use or keep the information. In Activity 3.8, we look at the readability and suitability of a health resource.

Activity 3.8   Critical thinking

Find a health education leaflet or booklet from your place of work that you might use with patients. Use the resources above to work out the readability and suitability of the resource.

As this activity is for your own assessment, no outline answer is provided.

Having completed Activity 3.8, you should now have a better idea of how to communicate health using a resource such as a pamphlet or leaflet. We will now look at electronic and online communication.

Electronic and online communication

Communication in nursing has developed and extended to using electronic formats. The most common format you will use is electronic mail (e-mail). Other areas used are Skype and FaceTime; some hospitals are using robots to assist in ward rounds. Another rapidly developing area is the use of social media for communication and professional purposes. First, however, let us look at the use of e-mail.

Communication using e-mail

E-mails are used more and more to communicate with patients and other colleagues; they also create an electronic trail. Some of the reasons for the growing use of e-mail for communication are: it is easy to use and there are economic advantages; it is a quick way to give information, updates and appointments; it is easy to recall if needed; it is reliable, secure and a good way to keep records of patient and staff communication. However, some rules need to be followed to ensure confidentiality, quality and secure communication. First, patient consent has to be obtained, especially if the communication will contain confidential and/or sensitive information. Your hospital will have an encryption service for e-mails sent outside the organisation. Make sure that the contact details are correct. E-mail communication should be written in a professional way. However, professional does not mean using technical jargon – the communication should be clear and easy to understand. Avoiding misunderstanding is really important – for example, only use upper-case letters where necessary as writing in upper-case can be interpreted as shouting or rudeness. Always provide the patient with an option to contact you if needed. This can be in the information contained in your e-mail signature. The electronic signature should be at the end of the e-mail and contain your full name, position, ward or department, hospital trust and phone contact with your e-mail. For confidentiality purposes, never leave your e-mail box open or unattended. The section Communicating with a patient using e-mail (below) is an example of how to write an e-mail to a patient.

- It is always good practice to start an e-mail with the person's name and a greeting.
- You should introduce yourself.
- Then write the actual information you want to provide the patient with, in the clearest way possible, avoiding jargon and acronyms.
- Formally end the e-mail with, for example, kind regards or best wishes, followed by your signature.

Remember to keep the e-mail simple and always offer support. Even by e-mail, patient data are still patient data. Confidentiality needs to be ensured and compliance with hospital data-handling policies has to be adhered.

Communicating with a patient using e-mail

Dear Ms Jones I hope this email finds you well. I am student nurse Xabi Cathala from Nightingale Ward at London South Bank Hospital.

I am writing to you to let you know that we have arranged an outpatient appointment for you on Tuesday, 16 December 2020. Your appointment time is 1400 (2pm). On arrival at the hospital, can you please report to the main reception and they will direct you to the Orthopaedic Outpatient Department.

To confirm your appointment or queries, please call on 0209 511 4567.

We look forward to seeing you.

Kind regards

Xabi Cathala

Student Nurse

Nightingale Ward

London South Bank Hospital

Phone: 0209 511 4567

E-mail: CathalaX@LSBH.net

Skype and FaceTime

Skype and FaceTime are digital technology that can be used for communicating with patients or colleagues in real time. You will need a computer or smart device such as a phone, tablet or iPad. An internet connection is needed; to use Skype, you will need to have an application downloaded to your device to enable the communication. When you are using this type of technology for communication, you will need to ensure that you maintain privacy and confidentiality. Activity 3.9 helps you identify how you can do this.

Activity 3.9   Critical thinking

1. Make a list of the situations you may use Skype or FaceTime to communicate with a patient.

2. Make a list of how you will maintain privacy and confidentiality when using Skype or FaceTime for patient communication.

An outline answer is provided at the end of the chapter.

Activity 3.9 will have helped you to identify the various ways you can communicate using real time. When you are using online communications, you should follow the same practice as if you were in a physical space. Therefore, you should ensure that privacy is maintained. You may do this by ensuring that you are using a room or office, with a door that you can close to keep conversations private. Ensure that no one else is able to hear you or see the patient you are communicating with. This is particularly important if it is a consultation in which the patient may be asked to expose their body. Ensure that you have consent to carry out the consultation online. As a first-year student nurse, you may not be asked to undertake take such a task, but you need to be aware of how to maintain privacy and confidentiality in such online communication.

Social media for professional nursing purposes

Social media is simply a collective of websites or online applications that allow individuals to communicate and network through sharing content. This content may be text, pictures or short videos. *The Code* (updated 2018) from the Nursing and Midwifery Council has provided clear guidance on how nurses should use social media. One of the statements in *The Code* is: *Use all forms of spoken, written and digital communication (including social media and networking sites) responsibly.* (*The Code*, paragraph 20.10). Before we look at responsible use of social media as part of communication, let us use the next activity to identify the main types of social media.

Activity 3.10   Critical thinking

Make a list of the different types of social media that you know.

An outline answer is not provided, but in the section below we identify some of the social media platforms that you may be familiar with.

There is an abundance of social media sites and applications. Some of the most common are Facebook, Twitter, Instagram, Pinterest, YouTube, Vimeo, Snapchat, LinkedIn and WhatsApp. Some of these are used for professional purposes – for example, the group @WeNurses is on Twitter and Facebook (there is also a @WeStudentNurses group). WeNurses provides professional content relating to nursing and healthcare, and have used social media to build an online nursing community (Moorley and Chinn, 2014). They hold weekly online real-time discussions on topics pertinent to nursing. Activity 3.11 gets you to look at the WeNurses website.

Activity 3.11   Critical thinking

Visit the WeNurses website at www.wecommunities.org/. Once you are on the web page, look at the calendar of chats and choose one to participate in. Look at the chats aimed towards students.

As this activity is for your own research, an outline answer is not provided.

You would have seen from Activity 3.11, WeNurses provides guidance and tips for tweeting. As a nurse, you must remember that your professional code of conduct (*The Code*) stipulates that you need to maintain patient privacy and confidentiality at all times (NMC, 2018). The golden rule in social media nursing communication is that if you would not say or do it offline, do not do it online. Put simply, do not make a post online if you would not do it in a face-to-face situation. You should also not post pictures of patients online and be mindful of taking photos to post online where patients' details may be captured unintentionally. Most National Health Service hospitals have a social media policy and you should familiarise yourself with this.

Patients and their families also use social media to communicate using post or direct messaging (DM). The next case study, continuing the story of Ms Jones, is designed to help you develop your communication skills when talking about social media.

Case study: Ms Jones (continued)

Later on, during your shift, Ms Jones from our first case study tells you that you are such a kind, caring and considerate nurse and that she is really glad you are the nurse caring for her. She goes on to tell you that she has looked you up on Facebook and sent you a friend request.

Let's think of how you could use indirect communication with Ms Jones regarding the above situation. First, you must remember your professional code of conduct (this was outlined in Chapter 1). It is best professional practice not to befriend patients on social media. You may begin by saying 'Thank you', then pause and say 'That's a lovely gesture, but my professional code of conduct does not allow me to engage with patients whose care is my responsibility'. You may also want to highlight that there are professional boundaries and you will be crossing these if you were to pursue a social media connection. As a student, you should acknowledge that in direct communication you send a clear message and the receiver (in this case, the patient) understands what you are delivering. You may want to practise this with one of your peers.

Social media should not be shunned and while there are negative examples associated with its use in nursing and healthcare, there are much more positive outcomes. There are numerous benefits to using social media as a student nurse and you will need to learn how to leverage this for your benefit. On Twitter there are student communities who are supporting each other in the learning environment. Ferguson et al., 2016 showed how first-year nursing students have used Facebook to make the transition to university. There are many opportunities to use social media for professional nursing communications and guidance is available to help you – for example, the Nursing and Midwifery Council produced guidance on how to use social media responsibly (see the Useful websites section at the end of the chapter for the weblink to access this resource).

Chapter summary

This chapter aimed to introduce you to the different types of communication and how you will use them in your professional career as a nurse. We have provided you with information on how to communicate with patients, including patients from different social backgrounds. This chapter has shown you how to deliver health promotion information and advice use, some simple do's and don'ts of how to communicate and how to use *The Code* in guiding your communication as part of your professional responsibility. In this chapter we have provided you with guidance on how to use electronic and online communication tools and applications. We have emphasised that patient confidentiality and privacy should be maintained at all times as we use new and emerging communication tools.

Activities: Brief outline answers

Activity 3.1   Critical thinking (p55)

The following are some of the ways in which you can communicate with the patient in the case study:

- Verbal: you can give information to the patient through talking.
- Reading materials: you may be able to communicate information about the ward through a leaflet or pamphlet.
- You can also use non-verbal communication such as nodding your head.
- As the patient has a smart device, you can also send e-mails or direct her to websites with relevant information.

Activity 3.4   Critical thinking (p59)

1. This will be applicable to your own culture but, for example, some cultures insist that you call the older person by a prefix such as Mr or Mrs. Other cultures may stipulate that you use a more friendly term such as uncle or aunty, or you may come from a culture where you can call the older person by their first name.

2. This will be based on your own cultural belief. However, some cultures may view mental health as a form of witchcraft or black magic.

3. The answer relies on your own beliefs and is personal to you.

Activity 3.6   Critical thinking (p62)

1. One of the social/environmental barriers could be exercising in a place where a person does not feel safe, or there might not be affordable facilities to continue exercising. Family commitment such as childcare or care of other relatives may impact on the ability to exercise and engage in physical activity.

   Facilitators may include community space for exercising that is well lit and has a supervisor. Local walking groups may help, as well as cooking groups in a community hall or after-work clubs.

2. This will be based on your knowledge of your local area. You can look at your local authority or council websites for helpful information.

Activity 3.7   Critical thinking (p64)

Some of the areas you may have identified as helpful are:

- The layout of the resource.
- The use of simple language.
- Short sentences.
- The use of images.
- The use of drawings that are not complex.
- The use of thumbs up and down.
- Good use of colours.

Activity 3.9   Critical thinking (p66)

The situations in which you may use Skype or FaceTime to communicate with a patient are, for example:

1. For a consultation on treatment advice or follow-up on how prescribed treatment is progressing.

2. To provide advice on medication or explain instructions on how to take prescribed medication.

Some key areas to note in maintaining privacy and confidentiality when using Skype or FaceTime for patient communication are:

1. Always ensure your connection is secure.

2. Ensure prior face-to-face contact with the patient before commencing Skype to confirm their identity.

3. Do not conduct the consultation in the presence of others without the patient's permission and take reasonable measures to avoid inadvertent disclosure of information.

4. Close the office door before initiating or receiving a Skype call and use signs to indicate that a consultation is taking place.

Some other points to note are: ensure that other staff members are aware that Skype is used for consultations within the clinic to minimise risk of unintended interruptions. Inform patients that Skype cannot protect users from spyware, which can compromise their security. Advise patients to ensure they have adequate anti-virus protection on their computers. Make patients aware that some personal information from their Skype account is stored locally on the computer. This is particularly important if patients intend to use public or shared computers. Advise patients to log out of their Skype account when not in use. Ensure that you are in an area that allows privacy and confidentiality to be maintained – for example, a closed room or dedicated consultation suite.

Further reading

Corcoran, N (2011) *Working on Health Communication.* London: SAGE.

Corcoran, N (ed.) (2013) *Communicating Health: Strategies for Health Promotion.* (2nd edn). London: SAGE.

Useful websites

Use this website to undertake Activity 3.6:

www.nhs.uk/change4life

This website provides information and tips for making lifestyle changes.

Use this website to undertake Activity 3.7:

www.macmillan.org.uk/

This website provides information on cancer and some answers to the fundamental questions you may have on the disease.

www.bhf.org.uk/

This website provides information on heart disease and some answers to the fundamental questions you may have on the disease.

www.ageuk.org.uk/

This website provides information on older people and the support available.

www.samaritans.org/

This website provides support for people who need someone to talk to about any problems they may be encountering.

WeNurses:

www.wecommunities.org

This is an online nursing community using social media applications.

Nursing and Midwifery Council:

www.nmc.org.uk/standards/

This is the regulator of nurses, midwives and health visitors in the United Kingdom.

Use this website to learn about Gerard Egan model of communication: **www.counsellingcentral. com/the-egan-model-and-soler/**

The Royal College of Nursing is a nursing union and provides support for social media usage in nursing:

www.rcn.org.uk/professional-development/publications/pub-004534

https://rcni.com/hosted-content/rcn/first-steps/why-communication-important

Use this website for guidance on safe use of social media: **www.nmc.org.uk/globalassets/ sitedocuments/nmc-publications/social-media-guidance.pdf**

Chapter 4

Professional skills for adult nursing

Part 1

Calvin Moorley and Alwin Puthenpurakal

NMC Standards of Proficiency for Registered Nurses

Platform 1: Being an accountable professional

Registered nurses act in the best interests of people, putting them first and providing nursing care that is person-centred, safe and compassionate. They act professionally at all times and use their knowledge and experience to make evidence-based decisions about care. They communicate effectively, are role models for others, and are accountable for their actions. Registered nurses continually reflect on their practice and keep abreast of new emerging developments in nursing, health and care.

At the point of registration, the registered nurse will be able to:

1.8 demonstrate the knowledge, skills and ability to think critically when applying evidence and drawing on experience to make evidence informed decisions in all situations;

1.16 demonstrate the ability to keep complete, clear, accurate and timely records;

1.17 take responsibility for continuous self-reflection, seeking and responding to support and feedback to develop their professional knowledge and skills;

1.20 safely demonstrate evidence-based practice in all skills and procedures stated in Annexes A and B.

Platform 2: Promoting health and preventing ill health

Registered nurses prioritise the needs of people when assessing and reviewing their mental, physical, cognitive, behavioural, social and spiritual needs. They use information obtained during assessments to identify the priorities and requirements for person-centred and evidence-based nursing interventions and support. They work in partnership with people to develop person-centred care plans that take into account their circumstances, characteristics and preferences.

At the point of registration, the registered nurse will be able to:

3.4 understand and apply a person-centred approach to nursing care, demonstrating shared assessment, planning, decision making and goal setting when working with people, their families, communities and populations of all ages

3.5 demonstrate the ability to accurately process all information gathered during the assessment process to identify needs for individualised nursing care and develop person-centred evidence-based plans for nursing interventions with agreed goals.

Platform 4: Providing and evaluating care

Registered nurses take the lead in providing evidence based, compassionate and safe nursing interventions. They ensure that care they provide and delegate is person-centred and of a consistently high standard. They support people of all ages in a range of care settings. They work in partnership with people, families and carers to evaluate whether care is effective, and the goals of care have been met in line with their wishes, preferences and desired outcomes.

At the point of registration, the registered nurse will be able to:

4.8 demonstrate the knowledge and skills required to identify and initiate appropriate interventions to support people with commonly encountered symptoms including anxiety, confusion, discomfort and pain.

Chapter aims

After reading this chapter, you will be able to:

- describe the essential and professional skills and knowledge that underpins professional nursing practice across the adult life span;
- identify the key issues in providing safe and high-quality care, including the assessment of pressure areas, nutrition, risk of falling, continence, track and trigger systems and the interventions to manage these conditions;
- develop and expand your knowledge, practical ability and professional attitudes in promoting high-quality care through embedded learning activities in this chapter;
- demonstrate awareness of reflection of your own values and beliefs, and how this may affect their interactions with patients their carers and families.

Introduction

This chapter starts with the case study below to illustrate the importance of essential clinical skills and knowledge in nursing. As an early student practitioner of nursing, you will experience a myriad of clinical scenarios. Almost all of these will require a thorough understanding of essential nursing skills, clear and concise documentation of assessments and the ability to apply evidence-based theory into clinical practice. Throughout this chapter, you will be introduced to the skills and knowledge underpinning common assessment methods and techniques used in most of the acute and continuing care settings.

Case study: Jo

After having an argument with her boyfriend, Jo (28 years old) ran away from her apartment. While running, she tripped and fell on the pavement, sustaining a small bruise to her knee. Two days later, she came down with a cold and the bruise on her knee looked very swollen. Despite self-medicating on over-the-counter pain-killers, she did not experience any improvement. She went to the local walk-in centre and a healthcare professional advised her to nurse herself at home with extra bandages and over-the-counter remedies. A week later, she was found collapsed in her home. Her boyfriend called the emergency services and without delay she was taken to her local accident and emergency department (A&E). On admission to the department, Jo looked pale and was clammy, drifting in and out of consciousness with shallow breaths and a weak pulse. Once in the emergency department, the team worked hard to figure out what caused her to collapse at home. They examined her and noticed that the bruise on her knee looked infected. Her knee showed signs of inflammation, she had a pyrexia, tachycardia and was hypotensive. She was drowsy and it was difficult to rouse her. An infection screen was undertaken which included blood cultures, a urine sample and wound swab, and these were sent for culture and sensitivity. An intravenous cannula was inserted and she was commenced on intravenous fluids and closely monitored by a staff nurse.

A first-year nursing student was shadowing the staff nurse who looked after Jo since her admission to A&E. She observed how carefully and systematically each and every member of the healthcare team worked to assess and care for her. The team treated her with a working diagnosis of sepsis. Jo needed to be nursed very attentively and was transferred to a high-dependency unit. The student nurse followed Jo to observe her patient journey. She noticed a range of assessments being carried out since Jo's first admission and an equal amount of documentation accompanied the assessments; some clinical skill-sets were transferrable, irrespective of the clinical setting. After a month-long rehabilitation and round-the-clock care, Jo made a successful recovery and was safely discharged home. The student nurse reflected on her experience, from the first day when Jo came into the hospital and all the care she had received.

The case study described above is an increasingly clinical concern globally. The growing rate of infections and disease transmission, increased risk of surgical infections, widespread prevalence of antibiotic resistance and associated poly-pharmacy have resulted in the increased incidence of super bugs in hospital and community settings.

What is sepsis?

Sepsis is when the body's response to infection causes injury to its own tissues and organs. It is commonly known as blood poisoning or septicaemia, but these terms are often used once the infection has started affecting the body's organs. Currently, there is no gold standard definition – over the years several literatures have struggled to define sepsis. The European Society of Intensive Care Medicine and the Society for Critical Care Medicine (Singer et al., 2016) agreed a new consensus definition of sepsis and its related clinical criteria (fig 1; Sepsis-33). The most important changes were:

- The terms 'SIRS' and 'severe sepsis' were removed.
- Sepsis is currently defined as life-threatening organ dysfunction caused by a dysregulated host response to infection.
- Organ dysfunction is defined in terms of a change in baseline SOFA (sequential organ failure assessment) score.
- Septic shock is defined as the subset of sepsis in which underlying circulatory and cellular or metabolic abnormalities are profound enough to increase mortality substantially.

Akin et al. (2018) defines sepsis as an organ dysfunction that is life-threatening due to dysregulated host response to infection.

The Centre for Disease Control and Prevention (2017) identifies four types of infections that are commonly linked with sepsis. These infections primarily affect organs such as the lungs (pneumonia), kidneys (urinary tract infection), skin (bacteria on skin) and gut (imbalance of bacteria in the gut). It also affects other organs when the patient is said to be in a state of 'septic shock'. Gram-negative bacterial agents such as *Acinetobacter* and *Klebsiella* contribute to more than half of the clinical cases identified as sepsis-causing pathogens (Gotts and Matthay, 2016).

Not all pathogens can cause sepsis because of protection from the natural body's complex immune mechanisms. However, if the body's natural immune response is overwhelmed by the pathogen, this has a greater potential to develop into a state of sepsis. The people who are most vulnerable and are most susceptible to a diagnosis of sepsis include the very young (under 1 year old), the elderly (over 75 years), people with chronic medical conditions and those with a weakened immune system (NICE, 2018). Chronic conditions that suppress the immune system – for example, HIV/AIDS, cirrhosis, asplenia and autoimmune disease have been identified in studies of patients with sepsis (Kaukonen et al., 2014).

Signs of sepsis

In the activity below, read about the signs of sepsis and make a list of what to look for in a patient with sepsis.

Activity 4.1   Evidence-based practice and research

Go to the NICE website listed under Useful websites at the end of the chapter and read the signs that are indicative of sepsis.

Now make a list of what you will look for in identifying sepsis in a patient.

An outline answer is provided at the end of the chapter.

Now that you have a better idea of identifying the signs of sepsis, we will look at patient assessment. In the following section we cover consent, and objective and subjective data collection.

Patient assessment

The main reasons for assessing a patient is that you can obtain a baseline in terms of clinical reading, develop a picture of the patient's ability to perform certain tasks, and determine the level of support required to maintain a safe recovery and environment. This initial assessment forms part of the risk assessment of the patient. It is important to understand that patients may be at risk of falls, pressure injury, malnutrition, deep vein thrombosis, self-harm and other mental health areas such as depression or suicide, and pain (these examples are not exhaustive). Levett-Jones et al. (2010) advise to use the five rights of clinical reasoning. They define clinical reasoning as a manner in which a nurse gathers cues and processes the information to arrive at an understanding of the patient's current problem, risk or situation. It concerns planning and implementing interventions, evaluating outcomes, and reflecting on and learning from the reasoning process. In essence, clinical reasoning is dependent upon the nurse's ability to gather:

- the *right* cues and
- to take the *right* action for
- the *right* patient at the *right* time and
- for the *right* reason.

Before undertaking any nursing assessment or procedure, it is important to understand the concept of consent. To gain consent from a patient is to seek permission. When you are going to assess or perform any task or a procedure that involves a patient, you will need to establish agreement beforehand. Informed consent is agreement with full knowledge of the possible consequences – i.e. any possible risks and the benefits. It acts to protect the autonomy of the patient by promoting meaningful collaborative decision-making between the health practitioner and the patient. Authorised informed consent procedures document a decision that is made voluntarily by the patient. There is no legal proxy consent by the next of kin in the UK unless the client has a lasting power of attorney. In the event that the person lacks capacity and does not have a legal advance directive of care that identifies their wishes, the clinician has to act in the patient's best interests (see Useful websites at the end of the chapter for consent guidance). This relies on the accuracy of the information given (which is done by you) and the capacity to interpret the information (by the patient or their next of kin). Acting in the best interest of the patient is echoed in *The Code* produced by the Nursing and Midwifery Council (NMC, 2018). It emphasises the significance of obtaining clear, informed consent by prioritising people and their wishes. As you familiarise yourself with *The Code*, you will see that it gives equal importance to correct documentation prior to initiating the consented task. Later in this chapter we discuss documentation and evaluating care. You may find that acquiring informed documented consent is a time-consuming process, but it is important to understand that the rights and interests of patients must be preserved when commencing any clinical task (Schenker et al., 2011).

Without assessment, the rest of the process, which includes planning care, implementing care and evaluating care, cannot take place. This is because a thorough holistic assessment determines the individual needs of the patient. Part of the assessment is concerned with the gathering of facts, which is also called objective information, and subjective information, which includes the patient's views, practice and rationale for their experience. After both types of data are collected, you can make a provisional diagnosis. An individualised, holistic, patient-centred data-collection method would assist any practitioner to pinpoint their decision-making process and deliver care tailored to specific patient needs. Another way of thinking of objective and subjective data is thinking about signs and symptoms. Signs would be your objective data – that is, what you are able to observe – and symptoms would be what the patient is telling you they are experiencing. For example, the patient may say they are shivering due to feeling cold; shivering will be a symptom of feeling cold, and when you take the temperature, the reading you get will be the sign that the patient is cold, hot or ambient temperature. The next activity asks you to look at objective and subjective patient data collection.

Activity 4.2   Critical thinking

For the first activity, Activity A, make a list of the objective data you will collect when assessing a patient.

For Activity B, make a list of the subjective data you will collect when assessing a patient.

An outline answer is provided at the end of the chapter.

Performing an assessment

To perform a successful assessment, the nurse must be able to use knowledge of basic physiology, pathophysiology and critical thinking skills. This can help you to formulate questions to enquire and be able to gather the most pertinent information so that the most appropriate care can be planned.

Assessment should not only include clinical measurements such as the patient's vital signs – e.g. heart rate or pulse, blood pressure, temperature, respiration rate, blood glucose levels, and height and weight, or similar primary data. It must also include secondary or subjective data such as what the patient is thinking, feeling, their fears and what help they may require during their stay in hospital.

Assessment should also focus on what may be needed on discharge (as ideally discharge of a patient begins on admission and assessment) such as community nurse visits, personal care assistance or home adaptions. A holistic assessment can also include such things as where the patient works, where the patient lives and other information regarding the patient's lifestyle. Conducting an assessment holistically is important because the patient's lifestyle has a direct impact on their health and on the nursing care they may require. For example, certain religions have beliefs that affect diet or have periods of fasting, so careful planning of care around the patient's diet would be essential. This may also affect how medication is delivered. Leisure activities may also influence a patient's overall health – for example, sport-related injury or risk of orthopaedic ailments.

In the case study above, Jo was found collapsed at her home. Her boyfriend consequently called the emergency services to request urgent help. The paramedics or emergency practitioners would have performed a short but concise assessment instead of a holistic assessment. The use of such assessment would be to determine immediate life-threatening needs such as the level of Jo's consciousness, maintenance of her airway, looking for signs of any obstruction that might affect her breathing, variations in her circulation and any neurological or external issues that might cause her to deteriorate.

To fully explore Jo's problems, the healthcare team at the hospital would have performed a holistic assessment. Her next-of-kin would be a useful resource in determining Jo's needs when she was in a state of poor health. This is carried out to obtain as much information as possible, not limiting to her physiological needs, but also valuing her psychological needs and expectations, including consent and health-related wishes.

The process of data collection via various types of assessments will continue after Jo's admission. This approach of 'continuous scanning for new knowledge' equips the clinical practitioner with a wealth of information to provide the best care possible for the patient. In the activity below, two types of commonly used assessments are described. A short and succinct assessment such as the Airway Breathing Circulation Disability

Exposure (ABDCE) approach, and comprehensive and continuous approach through the use of Roper–Logan–Tierney Model of Nursing based on daily activities. This is a theory-based assessment to see how the patient's life has been altered due to illness and hospital admission, and assesses independence and dependence on the activities of living. The activities of living identified by Roper et al. (2000) are:

- maintaining a safe environment;
- communication;
- breathing;
- eating and drinking;
- elimination;
- washing and dressing;
- controlling temperature;
- mobilisation;
- working and playing;
- sleeping;
- death and dying;
- expressing sexuality.

The next activity should help you to understand why certain types of assessments are used instead of others. It is anticipated that there is no one magic-bullet assessment that fits all scenarios, which is the same when caring for patients. Time and the patient's acuity are the key factors that will enable a clinical practitioner to choose between models of assessments in clinical practice.

Activity 4.3   Evidence-based practice and research

Using the information in the case study we presented at the beginning of the chapter, look at the assessments below and decide which is best suited and at which stages of the scenario you will use them. You can discuss your ideas with your colleagues and mentor. The web pages at the end of the chapter will assist you in finding the most suitable assessment, and we have also provided two journal articles that can assist you in understanding how these assessments are applied with a clinical caseload.

1.   *Short and succinct assessment practice*

The ABCDE approach

Go to Useful websites at the end of the chapter and, using link no. 2, read the ABCDE assessment.

(Continued)

(Continued)

Journal article

You should be able to access the articles below through your university's library; read these before starting this activity.

Cathala, X and Moorley, C (2019) A practical guide to completing an A–G assessment. *Nursing Times* (in press).

Thim, T, Krarup, NHV, Grove, EL, Rohde, CV and Løfgren, B (2012) Initial assessment and treatment with the Airway, Breathing, Circulation, Disability, Exposure (ABCDE) approach. *International Journal of General Medicine, 5*: 117.

2.   *Comprehensive and continuous assessment practice*

The Roper–Logan–Tierney model of nursing

Go to Useful websites at the end of the chapter, link no. 3, and read the Roper–Logan–Tierney model of nursing.

You should be able to access the article below through your university's library; read it as part of this activity.

Moura, GND, Nascimento, JCD., Lima, MAD, Frota, NM, Cristino, VM and Caetano, JA (2015) Activities of living of disabled people according to the Roper–Logan–Tierney model of nursing. *Northeast Network Nursing Journal, 16* (3).

Make a list of all the different assessment tools you have observed being used in practice.

An outline answer is provided at the end of the chapter.

Assessment tools

From the last activity, you will have gathered that a vast amount of assessment tools are used in nursing and some of these are specific to certain areas of nursing and you may hear colleagues describe these areas as their speciality. However, there are some tools that you will need to know about as these are useful in planning care for any patient.

In the next subsections we present a brief overview and explanation of these assessment tools and in the next chapter you will be given more in-depth information and activities that will help you to use these tools safely and appropriately.

Assessing risk of pressure ulcer formation

When thinking of pressure areas, most students will identify the buttocks as a pressure area. However, there are other pressures areas to consider.

Activity 4.4   Critical thinking

Make a list of all the areas you would consider when you are assessing a patient's pressure areas.

An outline answer is provided at the end of the chapter.

The Waterlow score is a common tool for pressure area/injury assessment. It was developed in 1985 by Judy Waterlow, a clinical nurse educator. The tool is easy to use and provides information on patients at risk of pressure area injury or ulcers. The assessment is divided into seven items:

1. Build/weight
2. Height
3. Visual assessment of the skin
4. Sex/age
5. Continence
6. Mobility and appetite
7. Special risk factors, this is divided into tissue malnutrition, neurological deficit, major surgery/trauma, and medication.

Each item is scored individually and calculated to give an overall score, which gives an indication of the patient's risk of pressure injury. Based on the total score, there are three at-risk categories: if a patient scores 10–14, they are indicated as 'at risk'; a score of 15–19 indicates 'high risk' and a score of 20 and above indicates 'very high risk'. Go to Useful websites at the end of the chapter and use link no. 4 to download the free Waterlow assessment for smart devices.

Nutrition

When undertaking a nutritional assessment, you will need to utilise a number of skills such as visual (observation), communication and knowledge of how the body works, which is physiology and anatomy. Several tools exist for assessing nutritional status, and a common tool you will encounter is the MUST (Malnutritional Universal Screening Tool). MUST is a tool used to identify adults who are undernourished, malnourished or at risk of malnutrition or obese. There are three sections:

1. Body mass index (BMI).
2. Weight loss.
3. Acute disease effect.

Each section is weighted, and you will need to add the score of each step to get a total, which will tell you the category of the patient. There are three risk categories based on the total score; if a patient scores 0 it is low risk; a score of 1 is medium risk and a score of 2 or more is high risk.

Risk of falling

The National Clinical Institute for Excellence (NICE) defines a fall as any event where the individual's final position is resting on the floor or a lower level from where they began without the loss of consciousness (NICE, 2015). FRAT (Falls Risk Assessment Tool) is a commonly used tool for assessing the risk of falls in older people by healthcare professionals. The assessment has two parts: Part 1 focuses on the risk of falls and is based on a total score of 20; patients are categorised as low risk at 5–11; medium risk at 12–15 and high risk at 16–20. Automatic high risk includes recent change in functional status and/or medications affecting safe mobility (or anticipated), or dizziness/postural hypotension. Part 2 is a risk factor checklist with yes or no answers. It covers vision, mobility, transfers, behaviours, activities of daily living, environment, nutrition, continence and other conditions. The assessments end with Part 3, which is a plan of action/care.

Pain assessment

Most people admitted to hospital will experience some level of pain or discomfort due to their condition or the interventions they have to undergo. There are a number of tools available to assess the levels and severity of pain. The Numeric Pain Rating Scale is commonly used in adult nursing. It is an 11-point scale where 0 indicates no pain and 10 indicates the worst pain experienced. Therefore, the higher the score the more severe the pain. This tool is very effective as it is simple to use, is verbal and can easily be translated. An example of another pain tool is the Abbey Pain Score (2004), which is useful to use with patients who have problems articulating their needs and includes those with dementia (McMahon et al., 2019). The scale is used while observing the patient. There are six questions to address: vocalisation, facial expression, change in body language, behavioural change, physiological change and physical change. Each question is scored 0–3 where 0 is absent (no pain), 1 mild, 2 moderate and 3 severe. The score for each question is added together. The final score is 0–2 no pain, 3–7 mild pain, 8–13 moderate pain and 14+ severe pain. The tool also asks the assessor to indicate whether the pain is chronic, acute or acute on chronic. Other tools include the PQRST (Provokes, Quality, Radiates, Severity and Time) and Visual Analogue scale. Go to Useful websites at the end of the chapter and use link no. 7 to read about these.

Track and trigger systems

Track and trigger assessments are those that help you to identify a deteriorating patient. In the UK, it is recommended that you use the National Early Warning Score

(NEWS2); the latest version was published in December 2017. It is based on an aggregate score derived from assessing six physiological areas. These areas are: respiration, oxygen saturation, systolic blood pressure, pulse rate, level of consciousness or new confusion and temperature. Each physiological parameter is assigned a score and the total score indicates whether the patient is deteriorating. If a patient requires supplemental oxygen to maintain their saturation, then an additional 2 points are added to the total score.

In this section we have given you a simple overview of some of the assessment tools you will encounter in your first year of nursing.

Evaluating care and accountability

The reason we evaluate care is to ensure that the care we deliver is appropriate, meets the needs of the patient and identifies how we can modify the care where needed. Evaluating the care that you provide is linked to accountability, which is highlighted in the NMC *Code* (Cathala and Moorley, 2019). *The Code* makes clear the nurse's role in delegated tasks and the level of accountability that he or she carries with the care administered (NMC, 2018). It is only through evaluating the care you provide that you will be able to determine if the care you provided has been effective. Ideally, the evaluation should take the patient's view into consideration. The next activity helps you to identify what you would look for when evaluating care.

Activity 4.5   Critical thinking

Think of what you would consider when evaluating a patient's care who had complained of pain on your assessment and, together with your mentor and the patient, you devised and implemented a care plan.

An outline answer is provided at the end of the chapter.

Reflection and communication
Reflecting on care

As a student nurse, it is important to reflect on your practice and develop the skills of reflection as this can help you to improve the care you provide and identify learning needs. Evaluating care seldom connects nor corresponds the viewpoints of the end user – that is, the patient. The provision of high-quality care is complex and multifactorial, and involves multidisciplinary working (Groenewegen et al., 2005). Your reflection should aim to connect and value the feedback from the patient and their carers.

Reflection of care provided to a patient is an essential part of care quality improvement, which consequently solves problems, empowers decision-making and builds knowledge collaboratively.

Reflecting on professional practice

In the case study at the start of this chapter, Jo would have had to undergo various assessments and interventions, her health being the main priority among healthcare professionals and her family. It is important that Jo's consent is gained so that information about her can be shared with her partner. You should also ensure that you communicate with Jo about her care, which is part of the nursing process. This maintains professionalism through provision of discussion on all aspects of an intervention; thereby, Jo and her partner have the informed knowledge to make decisions to support her recovery from sepsis. This may not always be possible, especially during the first the stages of her admission process when her level of consciousness may vary. If the patient is unable to give consent, the nursing and medical team would have acted in the best interests of the patient. The patient or the carer have the right to ask questions relating to any aspect of the care given, and should be involved in evaluating the care delivery process. Offering open-ended questions during discussions, identifying needs and expectations, and actively listening to the carer or family member, provides them with the reassurance and eventually helps in the process of documenting what was communicated, interpreted and discussed.

As a first-year nursing student, you are exposed to clinical practice, which involves communication with patients and their families, friends and careers, as well as the multidisciplinary team.

Effective communication is an important part of care evaluation. All health professionals are required to document their delivery of care, intended and unexpected outcomes. The quality of this process determines how consistent and effective care outcomes are met and delivered.

Keeping an accurate record of nursing care that is planned and structured to address the individual needs and expectations is the responsibility of the nurse providing the care. As student nurses, practising how to write accurate accounts of nursing documentation is part of a nurse's education and augments clinical practice. Nursing documentations act as evidence of care delivery. As healthcare evolves with the help of technology, the multidisciplinary interventions and communications request even more clarity and accuracy in record keeping (Cathala and Moorley, 2019). Documentation takes into account the stages of admission, diagnosis (medical and nursing), all interventions and evaluation (Tuinman et al., 2017).

It is important that you understand that documentation has a profound impact in maintaining high standards within nursing practice, care planning, practice development and service improvement. It is often a common practice to document with the use of clinical acronyms and terminologies to maintain consistency and efficiency. However, you need to be mindful that excessive use of institutional abbreviations is often linked with misinterpretations of documentation (Johnson et al., 2010). *The Code* (NMC, 2015) highlights the importance of clarity and accuracy of documentation and the compliance of such established standards.

Activity 4.6 Reflection

Use the questions in this activity to reflect on your clinical practice as a student nurse, and discuss the findings with your colleagues and mentor. You may also use the case study in this chapter for the purpose of reflection.

- What are the different types of evaluation you have come across in practice?
- How and what are we comparing the evaluation with?
- What are the practical issues to consider during nursing care evaluation?
- Should we do the evaluation of care ourselves, or who else is better to evaluate the care that you have given?
- How should we best communicate the findings from evaluation?
- What are the different types of documentations you have come across and what are they for?
- How can you improve your documentation skills?

As this is a reflective exercise, no outline answer is provided.

Communication and reflection

Professional skills, communication and reflection work concurrently with shared decision-making. Shared decision-making is considered one of the features of patient empowerment, the others being patient-centredness and self-determination (Castro et al., 2016). These are achieved through implementing good communication between nurses and patients. As a vital skill in nursing, good communication helps in all areas of nursing interventions, from prevention and treatment to rehabilitation and health promotion.

To help Jo recover, the nurse and the student nurse would have showed good professional rapport by asking and enquiring with kindness and empathy, showing interest in their activities of daily living and experiences, developing trust and confidence in each other, both patient and practitioner. This humanistic approach preserves the patient's welfare, values and dignity. Clear communication, promoting mutual respect, compassion and upholding basic human rights are founding pillars in established nursing practice of prioritising people (NMC, 2015).

Activity 4.7   Reflection

Consider the following scenarios and explore them with your understanding of skills in communication and reflection. Discuss your thoughts and answers with your colleagues and your mentor.

1. Mrs Brown is a retired schoolteacher and is anxious about her stay in hospital. She is also concerned about the pet she left at home. How can you help Mrs Brown feel less anxious in her new environment?

2. James's father has told you that 'James looks neglected by staff on the ward'. How will you approach this situation and ensure that both James and his father are in safe hands?

3. Think of a difficult moment in your clinical practice where you feel you were asked to undertake care that you have not been prepared for. How did you cope? What happened? Why do you think it happened? What could have been done to achieve a better outcome? How many different ways are there in which you can resolve this issue for a better outcome?

As this is a reflective activity, no outline answers are provided; however, we have discussed below how you can approach this activity.

In the last activity you would have approached question 3 in a reflective manner. Looking back at the past events and exploring this from all angles would have helped you to better comprehend and manage similar scenarios should they happen in the future. Through this question, you could use Gibbs' reflective cycle (1988).

By consciously thinking about your experiences and linking theory to practice, you would have practised the invaluable skill of being a reflective practitioner. Through this approach, you would have evaluated your personal and professional strengths and weaknesses, areas of excellence and improvement and, most importantly, areas of self-development as a student nurse. It is about recognising and understanding why a certain course of action was followed, how your knowledge and skills were used, and where can you see areas of professional and personal development.

Gibbs' model uses a simple approach, with six components: description, which asks you what happened; feelings, which focuses on what were you thinking and feeling at the time; evaluation, which is what was good and bad about the experience; analysis is where you focus on what sense you make of the evaluation; conclusion asks what else you could have done; action plan asks what you would do if this situation arose again. These simple questions enable you to identify what happened, why such events happened and what you can do in the future to make things better.

Reflection needs to be considered as a moment of rejuvenation in thinking. It can be immediate, called reflection in action, or latent, which is some time after the event. Student nurses should feel empowered and confident through reflection. As a professional skill, reflective practice goes hand in hand with communication, establishing professional standards, and valuing areas of learning and development in professional practice.

Chapter summary

The purpose of this chapter was to provide a brief introduction to professional skills in nursing. These skills include patient assessment, gaining consent and how to work as a team. It covered an overview of several assessments, including models of nursing care that you would most likely encounter in the first year of your nursing education and clinical practice. In this chapter, you were given activities on evaluation of nursing care and the importance of documenting care, as well as on communication and reflection as part of the professional skills you will need to develop in the first year of your student nursing practice.

Activities: Brief outline answers

Activity 4.1 Evidence-based practice and research (p76)

The risk factors according to NICE are listed below.

Risk factors for sepsis

Take into account that people in the groups below are at higher risk of developing sepsis:

- the very young (under 1 year) and older people (over 75 years) or people who are very frail;
- people who have impaired immune systems because of illness or drugs, including:
  - o people being treated for cancer with chemotherapy (see recommendation 1.1.9);
  - o people who have impaired immune function (for example, people with diabetes, people who have had a splenectomy, or people with sickle cell disease);
  - o people taking long-term steroids;
  - o people taking immunosuppressant drugs to treat non-malignant disorders such as rheumatoid arthritis;
- people who have had surgery or other invasive procedures in the past six weeks;
- people with any breach of skin integrity (for example, cuts, burns, blisters or skin infections);
- people who misuse drugs intravenously;
- people with indwelling lines or catheters.

Take into account that women who are pregnant, have given birth or had a termination of pregnancy or miscarriage in the past six weeks are in a high-risk group for sepsis. In particular, women who:

- have impaired immune systems because of illness or drugs (see recommendation 1.1.5);
- have gestational diabetes or diabetes or other comorbidities;
- needed invasive procedures – for example, caesarean section, forceps delivery, removal of retained products of conception;

- had prolonged rupture of membranes;
- have or have been in close contact with people with group A streptococcal infection – for example, scarlet fever;
- have continued vaginal bleeding or an offensive vaginal discharge.

Face-to-face assessment of people with suspected sepsis

- Assess temperature, heart rate, respiratory rate, blood pressure, level of consciousness and oxygen saturation in young people and adults with suspected sepsis.
- Assess temperature, heart rate, respiratory rate, level of consciousness, oxygen saturation and capillary refill time in children under 12 years with suspected sepsis. (This recommendation is adapted from NICE's guideline on fever in the under 5s.)
- Measure blood pressure of children under 5 years if heart rate or capillary refill time is abnormal and facilities to measure blood pressure, including a correctly sized blood pressure cuff, are available. (This recommendation is adapted from NICE's guideline on fever in the under 5s.)
- Measure blood pressure of children aged 5–11 years who might have sepsis if facilities to measure blood pressure, including a correctly sized cuff, are available.
- Only measure blood pressure in children under 12 years in community settings if facilities to measure blood pressure, including a correctly sized cuff, are available and taking a measurement does not cause a delay in assessment or treatment.
- Measure oxygen saturation in community settings if equipment is available and taking a measurement does not cause a delay in assessment or treatment.
- Examine people with suspected sepsis for mottled or ashen appearance, cyanosis of the skin, lips or tongue, non-blanching rash of the skin, any breach of skin integrity – for example, cuts, burns or skin infections – or other rash-indicating potential infection.
- Ask the person, parent or carer about the frequency of urination in the past 18 hours.

Activity 4.2   Critical thinking (p77)

Activity A: objective data:

- Demographic details such as age and gender.
- Clinical details such as blood pressure, pulse rate, temperature, respiration rate, blood glucose level. Any laboratory results that may be on file for the patient – for example, full blood count, electrolytes or imaging reports. The objective data is usually what you can observe.

Activity B: subjective data:

- How the patient is feeling – for example, this can be anxious, tired and/or low mood.
- The patient's experience of pain usually based on their pain threshold.
- The patient may self-diagnose based on what they have read on the internet.
- Complaints of symptoms related to how they feel – for example, coughing or itching.
- Reasons why they believe they are ill; this is often based on their beliefs and customs.

Activity 4.3   Evidence-based practice and research (p79)

The following list will be based on your placement experience – for example, if you were in a hospital or community setting, or acute or rehabilitation ward. This list is only an indication and is not exhaustive.

- Pressure injury tools – for example, Waterlow or Braden Scale.
- Consciousness level – for example, Glasgow Coma Scale.
- Nutrition assessment such as MUST (Malnutrition Universal Screening Tool).
- Infusion standards of practice assessing cannula sites for intravenous medication – for example, visual infusion phlebitis IVIP score.
- Manual handling assessment (may be individual to hospital).
- Oral/mouth assessment (may be individual to hospital).
- Pain: several tools exist – for example, numeric scale: 0 = no pain and 10 = worst pain.

Activity 4.4 Critical thinking (p81)

Some of the areas you will assess are:

- Ears: if a patient is positioned on their side, their ears may be comprised; also, wearing an oxygen mask or nasal cannula for an extended period of time can cause pressure injury. If the patient has a neckline such as a central venous catheter, they may lie on it and cause pressure injury.
- Elbows and any other bony parts such as the coccyx: bony areas may cause friction when rolling or turning a patient, or if a patient is sitting for a long period of time it can cause pressure injury.
- Buttocks: similar to the above, prolonged periods on the patient's buttocks can cause pressure injury.
- Heels: the patient's heels should be also be checked and assessed, as if they are wearing TEDS (anti-embolism stockings) these should be removed at least once per shift and the skin checked for shearing.

Activity 4.5 Critical thinking (p83)

- The areas you will want to consider when evaluating care are, overall, you will want to assess if the patient is pain-free or whether there has been a reduction in levels of pain experienced.
- After your initial assessment, you would have had a pain score from the patient, as well as the location and type of pain experienced. For example, the patient may have reported a pain score of 8 on the right side of his thigh, which is dull on rest but sharp on movement.
- Your intervention may have been to administer pain relief using the WHO analgesic ladder (see Useful websites, link no. 5). You may have also looked at changing the position of the patient and offering some sort of psychological intervention such as mindfulness.
- Based on your intervention(s), you will now evaluate the outcome. It is important to involve the patient in the evaluation. Some of the areas you will assess are asking the patient to score their pain using the same tool as you did on assessment; a reduction can indicate that the intervention is working. You may also want to ask the patient if repositioning helped and whether using mindfulness therapy was of any benefit.
- This evaluation shows the holistic approach to treating pain by considering areas other than pain medication.

Useful websites

1. Use this weblink to the National Institute of Clinical Excellence to compete Activity 4.1: **www.nice.org.uk/guidance/ng51**

2. Use this weblink to complete Activity 4.2: **www.resus.org.uk/resuscitation-guidelines/abcde-approach/**

3. Use this weblink to complete Activity 4.3: **www.nursing-theory.org/theories-and-models/roper-model-for-nursing-based-on-a- model-of-living.php**

4. Use this weblink to download the Waterlow assessment tool: **www.judy-waterlow.co.uk/index.htm**

5. Use this weblink to access the WHO analgesic ladder: **www.cpdconnect.nhs.scot/media/1698/controlofpaininadultswithcancer-11-appendices.pdf**

6. Use this weblink to read about patient consent: **www.nhs/uk?conditions/consent-to-treatment/**

7. Use this website to access reading on pain assessment tools: **www.evidence.nhs.uk/search?q=pain+assessment+guideline**

8. Use this weblink to read about sepsis: **www.survivingsepsis.org/Pages/default.aspx**

Chapter 5

Professional skills for adult nursing

Part 2

Calvin Moorley, Mynesha Sankar and Sonia Kirby

NMC Standards of Proficiency for Registered Nurses

Platform 1: Being an accountable professional

Registered nurses act in the best interests of people, putting them first and providing nursing care that is person-centred, safe and compassionate. They act professionally at all times and use their knowledge and experience to make evidence-based decisions about care. They communicate effectively, are role models for others, and are accountable for their actions. Registered nurses continually reflect on their practice and keep abreast of new emerging developments in nursing, health and care.

At the point of registration, the registered nurse will be able to:

1.8 demonstrate the knowledge, skills and ability to think critically when applying evidence and drawing on experience to make evidence informed decisions in all situations;

1.16 demonstrate the ability to keep complete, clear, accurate and timely records;

1.17 take responsibility for continuous self-reflection, seeking and responding to support and feedback to develop their professional knowledge and skills;

1.20 safely demonstrate evidence-based practice in all skills and procedures stated in Annexes A and B.

Platform 2: Promoting health and preventing ill health

Registered nurses prioritise the needs of people when assessing and reviewing their mental, physical, cognitive, behavioural, social and spiritual needs. They use information obtained during assessments to identify the priorities and requirements for person-centred and evidence-based nursing interventions and support. They work in partnership with people to develop person-centred care plans that take into account their circumstances, characteristics and preferences.

At the point of registration, the registered nurse will be able to:

3.4 understand and apply a person-centred approach to nursing care, demonstrating shared assessment, planning, decision making and goal setting when working with people, their families, communities and populations of all ages;

3.5 demonstrate the ability to accurately process all information gathered during the assessment process to identify needs for individualised nursing care and develop person-centred evidence-based plans for nursing interventions with agreed goals.

Platform 4: Providing and evaluating care

Registered nurses take the lead in providing evidence-based, compassionate and safe nursing interventions. They ensure that care they provide and delegate is person-centred and of a consistently high standard. They support people of all ages in a range of care settings. They work in partnership with people, families and carers to evaluate whether care is effective, and the goals of care have been met in line with their wishes, preferences and desired outcomes.

At the point of registration, the registered nurse will be able to:

4.8 demonstrate the knowledge and skills required to identify and initiate appropriate interventions to support people with commonly encountered symptoms including anxiety, confusion, discomfort and pain.

Chapter aims

After reading this chapter, you will be able to:

* explain the rationale for undertaking a patient assessment;
* demonstrate your understanding of systematic patient assessment;
* describe how assessments are undertaken using the relevant assessment tools;
* discuss assessment findings;
* identify when patient care should be escalated.

Introduction

In the previous chapter, a number of currently available assessment tools frequently used in clinical practice were identified. This was undertaken as a means to equip student nurses with the essential theoretical knowledge that underpins the provision of safe and high-quality, timely and holistic patient assessment in clinical practice. This chapter covers skin assessment, including the Waterlow score tool, and the SSKN (Surface, Skin, Keep, Incontinent, Nutrition) nutrition assessment tool – for example, Malnutrition Universal Screening Tool (MUST), the British Association Parenteral and Enteral Nutrition (BAPEN), the Confusion Assessment Method (CAM), the National Early Warning Score (NEWS), the Alert Confusion Voice Pain Unresponsive (ACVPU) assessment and the Situation Background Assessment Recommendation (SBAR) framework which is used to communicate patient information.

This chapter focuses on the application of key assessment tools in a systematic manner in order to improve and enhance patient care experience when adopting a holistic approach. This chapter will enable students to develop and expand on their problem-solving skills and highlights the importance of the nurse's role in escalating patient concerns through learning activities, as well as focusing on the professional values required of a healthcare professional in a complex healthcare environment.

The nursing process comprises four key areas: assessment, planning, intervention and evaluation. Patient assessment is one of the most important of these four pillars in the nursing process, without which patient care cannot be appropriately planned, implemented or evaluated. Much has been written about assessment in terms of collecting and analysing data about patients' physiological, psychological, sociocultural and lifestyles factors, which are the key to providing holistic care. Patient clinical assessment is sometimes difficult to implement in clinical practice, especially if the nurse is not familiar with the assessment tools available.

Numerous assessment tools have been developed in order to enable nurses to identify and articulate the needs of the patient so that appropriate care can be planned. It is worth noting that while these tools are there to assist in the identification of patients' needs, nurses should be mindful that an assessment tool is only as good as its user. Therefore, care must be taken to ensure that adequate training is provided for users so that when patient assessment is undertaken, it provides a holistic picture. In the case study below, Calvin is a student nurse who is learning how to undertake a skin assessment.

Case study: Calvin

Calvin is a student nurse on an oncology ward. He is working with his mentor, Steve, who has asked him to perform a skin assessment on a patient. The patient is a 56-year-old man, Winston, who has been having chemotherapy for his cancer of the lungs. Winston has been an inpatient for five weeks and has limited mobility, reduced appetite and has lost approximately 7kg since his admission to the ward. He is complaining that his skin is dry and itchy. Due to the effects of the chemotherapy, Winston is experiencing nausea and vomiting, and does not feel like eating much.

Before Calvin can start his assessment, he will need to demonstrate some knowledge of the skin and the assessment tool that Steve wants him to use.

Skin assessment

The skin is the first barrier that protects our body from potential infection. As we age, the skin loses its elasticity and has reduced skin turgor. The skin can become thin and translucent because of loss of dermis and subcutaneous fat. It then becomes dry and flaky because sebaceous and sweat glands are less active, due to the normal loss of peripheral skin turgor in the older adult. The breakdown of the skin due to, for example, reduced mobility, urine and faecal incontinence, poor dietary intake, damage caused by shearing and friction or a medical condition can contribute pressure injury. Therefore, a systematic assessment of the body is an important aspect of the nursing care of all patients. There are several assessment tools used within the clinical and community setting to systematically assess patients at risks. In Chapter 4, we discussed one of the more common tools, the Waterlow score which was developed by Judy Waterlow.

In Activity 5.1 we ask you to look at the skin.

Activity 5.1   Critical thinking

Draw a cross-section of the skin with it various parts. Try to label these parts.

An outline answer is provided at the end of the chapter.

A good understanding of the skin, as explored in Activity 5.1, is important when looking at pressure injury prevention among patients and there are various assessment tools to assist the nurse in assessing pressure injury.

Assessment tools

In order to identify, prevent and manage the pressure areas of all patients, there are a number of systems in place to assist the nurse to assess, implement and monitor care. These systems are useful in helping to determine when a nurse has some concerns whether to refer the patient to the medical and multidisciplinary team. Activity 5.2 asks you to consider the different skin assessments.

Activity 5.2   Research and evidence-based practice

When you are next on clinical placement, observe the various types of skin assessments that are undertaken. Discuss with your mentor why specific skin assessments are used. After this observation, do a literature search to identify the other types of pressure injury risk assessment tools available. Refer to Chapter 2 to see how to udertake a literature search.

As this activity is based on your own research, no outline answer is provided.

Having considered the various skin assessment tools in Activity 5.2, the next section focuses on how to assess the patient's skin using the Waterlow score assessment tool.

Using the Waterlow score tool

The Waterlow score tool was introduced in Chapter 4 and in this section we discuss how to use it.

Activity 5.3   Critical thinking

Steve has asked Calvin to undertake a skin assessment using the Waterlow score tool. How do you think Calvin should approach this assessment?

An outline answer is not provided as it is discussed in the sections below.

The primary aim of the Waterlow score tool is to assist the nurse to assess the risk of a patient/client developing a pressure injury. Most times, the nurse will use this tool together with clinical judgement.

The Waterlow score tool consists of seven items: build/weight, height, visual assessment of the skin, sex/age, continence, mobility and appetite, and special risk factors, divided into tissue malnutrition, neurological deficit, major surgery/trauma and medication.

The tool identifies three 'at risk' categories:

1.   a score of 10–14 indicates 'at risk';
2.   a score of 15–19 indicates 'high risk';
3.   a score of 20 and above indicates 'very high risk'.

For further information, see Useful websites at the end of the chapter, link no. 5 on how to perform a Waterlow score assessment.

SSKIN

The SSKIN Bundle Ulcer Prevention Tool (NHS Improvement, 2018) is a user-friendly document structured to implement and support the care management of patients who are at potential risk/or have developed a pressure ulcer. It is a standardised nursing skin assessment and care plan document. The form incorporates the Waterlow pressure ulcer assessment tool, a skin assessment with descriptions of different types of wound or skin conditions, the Malnutrition Universal Screening Tool Score and the skin care plan. For guidance on how to complete a SSKIN assessment, see Useful websites, link no. 2.

The mnemonic SSKIN stands for: Surface, Skin, Keep, Incontinent and Nutrition.

Surface: make sure your patient has the right support. A surface will be the areas you consider and you should look at the type of mattress the patient is lying on. For example, is it a foam or air mattress? If they are sitting on a chair, then the type of cushion the patient is sitting on will have to be assessed. These different surface types help to minimise pressure injury.

Skin inspection: assessment using an approved tool and regular assessment of the skin. As discussed, it is important to be familiar with the various types of skin assessment tools. A sound knowledge of the skin is also needed to know what to look for when carrying out an inspection.

In 2016, the National Pressure Ulcer Advisory Panel (NPUAP) changed using the term 'pressure ulcers' to 'pressure injury' and with this its definition was revised. The revised definition of a pressure injury is described as the injuries that usually occur over a bony prominence or under a medical or other device (Edserbg et al., 2016). They further explain that the injury can present as skin that is intact or an open ulcer that may be painful. The injury occurs as a result of intense and/or prolonged pressure or pressure in combination with shear. The tolerance of soft tissue for pressure and shear may also be affected by microclimate, nutrition, perfusion, co-morbidities and condition of the soft tissue.

There are four stages on the NPUAP webpage:

Stage 1 Pressure injury: non-blanchable erythema of intact skin. Intact skin with a localised area of non-blanchable erythema, which may appear differently in darkly pigmented skin. Presence of blanchable erythema or changes in sensation, temperature or firmness may precede visual changes. Colour changes do not include purple or maroon discoloration; these may indicate deep tissue pressure injury.

Stage 2 Pressure injury: partial-thickness skin loss with exposed dermis. The wound bed is viable, pink or red, moist and may also present as an intact or ruptured serum-filled blister. Adipose (fat) is not visible and deeper tissues are not visible. Granulation tissue, slough and eschar are not present. These injuries commonly result from adverse microclimate and shear in the skin over the pelvis and shear in the heel. This stage should not be used to describe moisture associated skin damage (MASD), including incontinence-associated dermatitis (IAD), intertriginous dermatitis (ITD), medical adhesive-related skin injury (MARSI) or traumatic wounds (skin tears, burns, abrasions).

Stage 3 Pressure injury: full-thickness skin loss. Full-thickness loss of skin, in which adipose (fat) is visible in the ulcer and granulation tissue and epibole (rolled wound edges) are often present. Slough and/or eschar may be visible. The depth of tissue damage varies by anatomical location; areas of significant adiposity can develop deep wounds. Undermining and tunnelling may occur. Fascia, muscle, tendon, ligament, cartilage and/or bone are not exposed. If slough or eschar obscures the extent of tissue loss, this is an unstageable pressure injury.

Stage 4 Pressure injury: full-thickness skin and tissue loss. Full-thickness skin and tissue loss with exposed or directly palpable fascia, muscle, tendon, ligament, cartilage or bone in the ulcer. Slough and/or eschar may be visible. Epibole (rolled edges), undermining and/or tunnelling often occur. Depth varies by anatomical location. If slough or eschar obscures the extent of tissue loss, this is an unstageable pressure injury (NPUAP, 2016).

Always start by looking at the skin from head to toe, identify any stage of pressure injury that may be present and find out if there are any factors that may predispose the patient to pressure injury. When inspecting the skin, pay special attention to:

1. the skin beneath and around any devices (e.g. cannulas) or compression (TEDS) stockings;
2. bony prominences (e.g. heels, sacrum, occiput);
3. skin-to-skin areas, such as the penis, back of knees, inner thighs and buttocks;
4. all areas where the patient may have limited sensation to feel pain;
5. areas in particular where they may have had a breakdown previously and there is scar tissue.

Be mindful if the patient is getting epidural/spinal pain medicines that may reduce skin sensation. It is good practice to consider the following five areas when assessing the skin: temperature; turgor (firmness); colour; moisture level and skin integrity – i.e. is the skin intact or are there open areas (breakages) or rashes that comprise skin integrity? (See Useful websites, link no. 1.)

Keep your patient moving. Mobility will help reduce the risk of skin damage and subsequent pressure injury. Encourage the patient as follows:

1. Do what they can for themselves, as long as they can do it safely. Public Health England (2018) has provided some guidance on prevention, which may include showering, dressing and walking to the toilet.

2. Walk around the ward every few hours if they are able to. If the patient has been advised not to walk by themselves, advise them to change their position every one to two hours, particularly moving their legs and ankles.

3. Whenever possible, encourage the patient to sit out of bed rather than sitting up in bed (sitting up in bed puts pressure on their tailbone or coccyx).

4. Move as frequently as possible. Explain that small changes in how the patient sits or lies can make a difference to reducing injury to the skin.

Incontinent, or moisture: ensure the skin is cared for correctly. The skin can break down and experience damage due to moisture. Assess if the patient's skin is frequently moist with urine or faeces (one or both). If the answer is yes for only one or both, then check the following:

1. Complete a full continence assessment. You should establish the cause of the faecal continence. Consider if you need to send a stool sample for to confirm infection.

2. Ensure the patient is toileted regularly.

3. Reassess the patient's continence status.

4. If the patient is using any aids such as pads and pants or urinary sheath or indwelling catheter, ensure they are worn and fit correctly.

5. Consider if pads need to be changed more often.

6. Cleanse the moist area of skin with water only and clean cloths.

7. Do not use soap; if necessary, the area can be cleaned with appropriate cleanser or emollient.

8. Apply a non-sting barrier cream or film and durable barrier creams. These would be prescribed by the medical team and dispensed by the pharmacy.

Nutrition: ensure good nutritional and oral fluid intake; the nutritional status of the patient is paramount to the health of their skin and its ability to heal if there is damage. The following should be performed as part of the assessment (you should do this with your mentor).

- All patients will be screened at first contact. The recommended tool for this is the Malnutrition Universal Screening Tool (MUST).
- Using MUST guidance, refer to a doctor or appropriate healthcare professional for nutritional support if indicated.
- Always remember that risk assessment should support, not replace clinical judgement.
- When considering any weight loss, perform a visual assessment of the patient. Look at clothing, jewellery and dentures as part of the assessment. Ask if their clothes, jewellery or dentures are looser, as this can indicate weight loss.
- Observe the patient's skin state and oral mucosa for signs of dehydration.

- Provide practical advice on nutritional support to improve dietary intake. Ensure that this is in line with the hospital policy. You can also provide health promotion materials such as leaflets on nutrition information.
- All patients with any pressure injury should be referred to dietetic services.

The aim of nutrition screening is to identify patients who are at risk from malnutrition or who are malnourished. The assessment also helps to identify the amount of nutrients that a patient may require and helps you to make appropriate recommendation(s). On assessment, information is usually collected on the patient's change in weight, body mass index or weight history, the ampleness of food intake and, with some tools, the severity of disease. Examples of two commonly used nutritional screening tools are the Malnutrition Universal Screening Tool (MUST) and the British Association Parenteral and Enteral Nutrition (BAPEN), which are discussed in the next section.

Malnutrition Universal Screening Tool (MUST)

To complete a MUST assessment, five steps need to be undertaken. You may not be asked to do this in your first year, but you should try to understand how to undertake the assessment.

Step 1: Measure height and weight and calculate the patient's BMI (Body Mass Index) score.

Step 2: Note the recent percentage weight loss and score. The MUST assessment tool will provide a table with the score for the related percentage loss.

Step 3: Establish the acute disease effect score.

Step 4: Add the scores from steps 1, 2 and 3 together to obtain an overall risk of malnutrition.

Step 5: Use management guidelines and/or local policy to develop a care plan.

British Association Parenteral and Enteral Nutrition (BAPEN)

Poor nutrition, reduced resistance to infection, dry and flaky skin, impaired wound healing, all increase the likelihood of muscle wasting. This can lead to a weak effort at mobilisation. Poor nutrition and hydration can also contribute to hypotension, causing dizziness and increasing the risk of falls. The nurse may be the first to notice signs of poor nutritional consumption, such as reduced fluid or dietary intake, leading to signs of malnutrition. Therefore, the nurse should reassess the patient and communicate their findings to the appropriate healthcare professionals, such as the dietitian. Activity 5.4 asks you to think critically about what you will do after you assess a patient for nutritional intake.

Activity 5.4 Critical thinking

Calvin has been asked to assess Winston from the case study at the beginning of the chapter. He has scored 2 on the MUST. What should Calvin do with the assessment findings? What documents/forms does he need to complete? How should Calvin hand over this information to other members of the multidisciplinary team?

An outline answer is provided at the end of the chapter.

Understanding how to communicate your findings to the wider team of healthcare professionals helps to identify the factors associated with pressure injury.

Risk factors associated with the potential of breakdown of pressure areas

When conducting skin inspection, follow your local guideline. An initial assessment must be done as close as possible to when the patient arrives on your ward or your first visit to their home setting in the community. It is possible to carry out a daily skin inspection when attending to personal hygiene, elimination needs or repositioning.

Remember that you need to gain consent from the patient, as this is an assessment to inspect all their skin for signs of pressure ulcers. Explain to the patient the reason why the assessment needs to be undertaken.

* Inspect the skin for colour, moisture, turgor. Note any bruising, redness, swelling and rashes. If there is an area of redness (erythema), gently press for 3 seconds; it should blanch and the colour return once you remove your finger. If the area remains white, this indicates pressure damage in the underlying tissue. In darker pigmented skin, it is more difficult to identify erythema and oedema; the change in tissue consistency is an important indicator of pressure damage in a dark skin tone.
* Care of patients at risk consists of a daily skin inspection. Those patients who are incontinent are at increased risk of developing moisture lesions. Moisture lesions are stage 2 pressure injury. It is skin damage that occurs as a result of excessive moisture from urine and/or faeces (Crook et al., 2014). Providing good hygiene care and barrier cream for patients who are incontinent is important, as well as regular repositioning to reduce localised pressure. As a nurse, you should encourage mobilising of patients every few hours; for those in their own home, you can set exercises that they can do in a chair or seated position. You can ask the physiotherapist for advice. It is important to speak to patients about good nutritional intake while in hospital and at home.

Resources and equipment

If a patient is unable to reposition themselves independently, healthcare professionals need to assist by either rolling the patient from side to side, or using appropriate equipment to assist – for example, sliding sheets. If a patient's assessment indicates that they are at risk of breakdown of pressure areas, a high-specification mattress should be used. These are usually mattresses that have an airflow system that helps to reduce pressure that can occur from immobility and the inability to reposition independently. Heel-protection pads also help to prevent injury on the heels. If the patient sits out, pressure support cushions may be necessary to reduce pressure on bony prominences such as the coccyx and aid comfort.

Multidisciplinary team

Involving other members of the multidisciplinary team in the care of the patient who is at risk or who has developed a pressure injury is vital. Following local guidelines and policies to liaise with other professionals for their intervention is part of the nurse's role to ensure that patients are referred to appropriate care services. As a nurse, you can liaise with the physiotherapist to promote mobility and assess for the appropriate equipment to prevent falls and encourage early mobilisation. The nurse can also refer the patient to the tissue viability team if the patient was admitted onto the ward with a stage 3 pressure injury or has developed a grade 3 pressure injury, for the correct treatment plan to promote healing. The dietitian/nutritional nurse may need to be contacted if the patient is losing weight or not eating. The dietetic team can undertake an assessment on what nutritional supplements the patient may need to prevent breakdown of the skin or promote healing of pressure ulcers. The doctor would also need to be informed if the patient has developed a pressure ulcer as an inpatient or has been admitted with an ulcer.

Documentation

The recording and documentation of a patient's repositioning is important. Each time a patient is repositioned, this should be recorded on the turning/SSKIN bundle chart to document as part of the nursing care evaluation.

Fall prevention

Falls in England in 2013 were the leading cause of injury and the ninth highest cause of disability-adjusted life years (DALYs) (Public Health England, 2018). This report also states that short- and long-term outlooks for patients are generally poor following a hip fracture, with an increased one-year mortality of between 18 and 33 per cent, and negative effects on daily living activities such as shopping and walking. It also highlights that falls in hospitals are the most commonly reported patient safety incident, with more than 240,000 reported cases in acute hospitals and mental health trusts in England and Wales. For older people, falls and fall-related injuries are a common and serious problem. The highest risk of falling is in people aged 65 and older, with 30 per cent of people older than 65 and 50 per cent of people older than 80 falling at least once a year (NICE, 2015a). NICE also reports that the cost to the NHS from falls is estimated to be more than £2.3 billion per year.

Although most falls do not result in serious injury, the consequences for an individual falling or not being able to get up after a fall can include psychological problems – for example, a fear of falling and loss of confidence in being able to move about safely, loss of or reduced mobility, leading to social isolation and depression, increase in dependency and disability, pressure-related injury and infection.

Standardised assessment tools are used to identify those patients who may be at risk of falling. All patients should be assessed upon admission for risk of falls. Below is a set of questions you can use when considering falls in patients.

1. Is the patient's admission to hospital related to a fall?
2. Has the patient had a fall in the last year?
3. Has the patient had an inpatient fall during this current admission?
4. Is the patient aged over 50 years with comorbidities that predispose to a fall or aged 65 years and over?
5. Does the patient need assistance with walking and transferring?
6. Is the patient experiencing any dizziness?
7. Does the patient exhibit any signs of confusion/agitation?
8. Does the patient have increased frequency of toilet usage?

Activity 5.5 is based on reflecting on the fall-prevention plans you may have encountered so far in your nursing career.

Activity 5.5   Reflection

Think about the various clinical areas you have worked on, including the community setting. What fall-prevention plans were put in place to prevent and reduce falls?

An outline answer is provided at the end of the chapter.

NHS Improvement has several resources that can help with falls prevention. Go to Useful websites at the end of the chapter, link no. 6, and read about these.

The next section focuses on the following assessments: Confusion Assessment Method (CAM); level of consciousness using ACPVU; National Early Warning Score (NEWS); Situation Background Analysis Recommendation (SBAR); WHO surgical checklist.

Confusion Assessment Method (CAM)

The Confusion Assessment Method is used to assess delirium in patients. The screening tool has four areas or features:

1. looks at acute onset and fluctuating course;
2. focuses on inattention;
3. assesses disorganised thinking;
4. focuses on altered level of consciousness.

Based on Nouye et al., 1990, below is an example of what the CAM looks like. Bear in mind that some hospitals may adapt this to suit their area.

Feature 1: acute onset and fluctuating course

The information on this feature is generally obtained from a family member or nurse and is demonstrated by positive responses to the following questions:

- Is there evidence of an acute change in mental status from the patient's baseline?
- Did the (abnormal) behaviour fluctuate during the day? This means did it come and go, or increase and decrease in severity?

Feature 2: inattention

This feature is shown by a positive response to the following question:

- Did the patient have difficulty focusing their attention – for example, were they easily distracted or did they have difficulty keeping track of what was being said?

Feature 3: disorganised thinking

This feature is shown by a positive response to the following question:

- Was the patient's thinking disorganised or incoherent – for example, was the patient rambling or was there irrelevant conversation, unclear or illogical flow of ideas, or unpredictable switching from one subject to another?

Feature 4: altered level of consciousness

This feature is shown by any answer other than 'alert' to the following question:

- Overall, how would you rate the patient's level of consciousness? Alert (normal), vigilant (hyper-alert), lethargic (drowsy, easily aroused), stupor (difficult to arouse), or coma (unarousable).

If features 1 and 2 and either 3 or 4 are present, it indicates that the patient is CAM +/ positive and a diagnosis of delirium is recommended.

Alert Confusion Voice Pain Unresponsive (ACVPU)

Alert Confusion Voice Pain Unresponsive is a scale used to measure levels of responsiveness. The assessment can only have one outcome for the five areas assessed. ACVPU is part of the National Early Warning Score 2 (NEWS2) assessment.

1. **Alert** If the patient is fully awake (note that they may not be orientated), their eyes will open spontaneously.

2. **Confusion** Confusion recognises any new state of confusion the patient may have. It excludes any pre-existing confusion that may arise from some illnesses such as dementia. It was added and updated in 2017 in NEWS2 to recognise any new confusion in the patient's status.

3. **Voice** In this part of the assessment, if the patient makes some sort of response when you talk to them, it means that they respond to voice or verbal command. This could be through opening their eyes when you speak to them, or by voice which may only be as little as a grunt, or it could be by moving a limb when asked to do so by the nurse or healthcare professional.

4. **Pain** A patient may respond to pain stimulus through their eyes (opening), voice (sounds) or movement (limbs). There are recognised ways for causing painful stimuli – for example, the trapezius squeeze which involves gripping and twisting a part of the patient's trapezius muscle. A patient who is fully conscious will locate the pain and make attempts to push it away, whereas a patient who is not alert and not responsive to a voice may only manifest involuntary flexion or extension of a limb.

5. **Unresponsive** This outcome is noted if the patient does not give any eye, voice or motor response to a voice or pain assessment.

If an ACVPU assessment score is less than alert (A), this is an indication that you may need to get further help. Below are some treatment options you can apply if the ACVPU is less than A.

- If the patient's conscious level is below A, seek medical help.
- Monitor the patient's level of response until help arrives.
- An unconscious patient is serious and the priority here is the patient's airway.
- Ensure that you maintain the airway patency.
- Place the patient in the recovery position.
- Treat any bleeding or cover open fractures.
- If available, administer oxygen therapy (this should be prescribed, but in an emergency situation you can administer oxygen without a prescription). Place pulse oximeter on the patient's finger and take a reading; if it is below 94 per cent, place the patient on oxygen therapy.

National Early Warning Score (NEWS2 updates 2017)

The National Early Warning Score is a simple aggregate scoring system in which a score is allocated to a physiological parameter. It is a track-and-trigger system to detect early deterioration in patients. The National Institute for Clinical Excellence (NICE) 2007 recommended that the parameters measured should be heart rate, respiratory rate, systolic blood pressure, level of consciousness, oxygen saturation and temperature. In 2017, it was updated and confusion was added to the level of responsiveness; two points were added to the final score if the patient requires supplemental oxygen.

A patient can gain a score of 0–3 (where 0 is good and 3 is cause for concern) in each physiological parameter. Figure 5.1 shows the NEWS2 chart with its scoring system.

The chart is shaded to show critical to non-critical levels. The shading provides both visual and numeric prompts to assist with identifying clinical parameters that are outside of the NEWS2 range.

Physiological parameter	Score						
	3	2	1	0	1	2	3
Respiration rate (per minute)	≤8		9–11	12–20		21–24	≥25
SpO$_2$ Scale 1 (%)	≤91	92–93	94–95	≤96			
SpO$_2$ Scale 2 (%)	≤83	84–85	86–87	88–92 ≤93 on air	93–94 on oxygen	95–96 on oxygen	≥97 on oxygen
Air or oxygen?		Oxygen		Air			
Systolic blood pressure (mmHg)	≤90	91–100	101–110	111–219			≥220
Pulse (per minute)	≤40		41–50	51–90	91–110	111–130	≥131
Consciousness				Alert			CVPU
Temperature (°C)	≤35.0		35.1–36.0	36.1–38.0	38.1–39.0	≥39.1	

Figure 5.1   NEWS 2 chart

Based on the aggregate score of the six parameters, the Royal College of Physicians (RCP) (2017) has recommended the following level to the trigger (score):

- *Low* score: an aggregate *new* score of 1–4.
- A single score of 3: an extreme variation in an individual physiological parameter (a score of 3 in any one parameter, which is the darkest shade on the NEWS2 chart).
- *Medium* score: an aggregate *new* score of 5 or 6. A *new* score of 5 or more is a key threshold and is indicative of potential serious acute clinical deterioration and the need for an urgent clinical response.
- *High* score: an aggregate *new* score of 7 or more.

The RCP (2017) has also made recommendations on how to respond to the triggers. Please see the points below for the actions to the level of trigger.

- A low *new* score (1–4) should prompt assessment by a competent registered nurse or equivalent, who should decide whether a change to frequency of clinical monitoring or an escalation of clinical care is required.
- A single score of 3 (the darkest shade – 3 in a single parameter) is unusual, but should prompt an urgent review by a clinician with competencies in the assessment of acute illness (usually a ward-based doctor) to determine the cause, and decide on the frequency of subsequent monitoring and whether an escalation of care is required.
- A medium *new* score (5–6) is a key trigger threshold and should prompt an urgent review by a clinician with competencies in the assessment of acute illness – usually a ward-based doctor or acute team nurse, who should urgently decide whether escalation of care to a team with critical care skills is required – i.e. critical care outreach team.
- A high *new* score (7 or more) is a key trigger threshold and should prompt emergency assessment by a clinical team/critical care outreach team with critical care competencies. Usually, this will also prompt the transfer of the patient to a higher dependency care area.

Activity 5.6 asks you to look at how to undertake and score the NEWS assessment.

Activity 5.6   Research and evidence-based practice

The Royal College of Physicians has provided an e-learning programme on NEWS2. Go the to the website https://news.ocbmedia.com/ and register to undertake the learning.

As this is an e-learning activity, no outline answer is provided.

From the e-programme in Activity 5.6, you will have learnt about raising an SBAR, which is discussed in the next section.

Situation Background Assessment Recommendation (SBAR)

If your patient has triggered a score that required medical attention, you will be required to raise an SBAR.

S – Situation

B – Background

A – Assessment

R – Recommendation

The SBAR is a communication tool that uses a set of standardised prompts to allow staff to share focused information in a concise and systematic manner. It is made up of four sections that are structured in a way that allows the individual to provide clear and relevant information that is reliable. The design of the SBAR helps to remove surplus information.

Activity 5.7 describes how to use an SBAR. In this activity, the four sections of the SBAR are provided with a scenario and you are then asked to practise communicating the information for each section.

Activity 5.7   Critical thinking

In this section of the tool, as the nurse you will need to do the following three actions:

- Identify yourself and the ward or site you are calling from.
- Identify the patient by name and state the reason for your call.
- Describe your concern.

An outline answer is given in the text below.

Scenario

Calvin is a student nurse and caring for Winston, who is in side room B on Anderson ward. Winston suddenly became short of breath and his oxygen saturation dropped to 86 per cent on room air, his respiration rate is 24 breaths per minute, heart rate 110 beats per minute and blood pressure 87/55 mmHg. His temperature is 38.7°C.

Together with his mentor, Steve, they have given Winston 5 litres of oxygen and his saturations have increased to 91 per cent, but his respiration rate remains high, ranging between 24 and 27. Calvin can see Winston using his accessory muscles to help his breathing. His chest sounds are not clear and you can hear an expiratory wheeze. He is alert on the ACVPU.

Using the three prompts in the situation below, raise this section of the SBAR.

Below is an outline answer.

Situation

I am Calvin Robert, a student nurse on Anderson ward.

I am calling about my patient Winston Johnson in side room B.

I am calling because I am concerned that his oxygen saturations have dropped to 86 per cent on room air and his respiration rate is 24bpm. His blood pressure is low, with a high heart rate and temperature.

Together with my mentor, we have placed him on 5 litres of oxygen and his oxygen saturations are now 91 per cent, but he is still working hard to maintain his breathing.

Background

You will need to provide the background to the situation. The following three prompts should be used.

- Provide the reason for the patient's admission.
- Explain any significant medical history.
- Inform the receiver of the information of the patient's background: admitting diagnosis, date of admission, prior procedures, current medications, allergies, pertinent laboratory results and other relevant diagnostic results.

For this part in the process, you need to have collected information from the patient's chart and notes.

Using the three prompts in the situation, raise this section of the SBAR. You may want to return to the initial scenario at the beginning of the chapter.

Below is an outline answer.

Answer

Mr Winston Johnson is a 56-year-old gentleman who was admitted five weeks ago (give the date) for chemotherapy. He had a diagnosis of cancer of the lungs in 2019. This is his fifth week of chemotherapy. He has bloods done every three days to check his haemoglobin, white blood cells and markers for sepsis and his last test shows (read the blood results to the receiver). Mr Johnson's condition has changed in the last 15 minutes. His last set of observations were: temperature 38.7°C, heart rate 110, BP 87/55 mmHg respiration rate 24–27bpm, oxygen saturations 91 per cent on 5 litres O_2. He is seen by the physiotherapist daily and has not needed any supplemental oxygen until now. Mr Johnson is alert.

Assessment

You need to think critically when informing the receiver of your assessment of the situation. Therefore, you will need to consider what might be the underlying reason for your patient's condition. This is where you need to connect your knowledge of anatomy and physiology, and how disease can affect the body's homeostatic mechanism. You have to take a global approach to your findings from your assessment to consolidate these with other objective indicators, such as laboratory results and X-rays, and any other relevant investigation results.

Under assessment, the following three prompts should be considered:

- Vital signs: look at the observations. What has changed? Is this change an improvement or a deterioration?
- Connections of pattern: here you need to try to think what is happening to your patient. This connects to the next point.
- Clinical impressions, concerns: based on your assessment and the patient's narrative, you need to make a provisional diagnosis – i.e. what you think is happening. You may not have an answer or impression; if this is the case, you need to communicate this.

Using the three prompts, raise the assessment part of the SBAR.

An outline answer is provided below based on the scenario.

Answer

I think the problem is respiratory distress secondary to the chemotherapy treatment. I have given 5 litres of oxygen via a face mask. I have repositioned the patient to assist with his breathing and reassured him. I have commenced regular observations.

If you are unable to make an impression, you can say:

I am not sure what the problem is, but Mr Johnson is deteriorating; *or* I don't know what's wrong, but I am really worried and would like you or one of your colleagues to come and review the patient.

Recommendation

This is the final part of the assessment communication. Here you will be able to make your recommendation.

- What you would like to happen by the end of the conversation. Any advice or specific request that is given on the phone needs to be repeated back to the speaker to ensure accuracy.
- The nurse should also explain what is required and be specific about request and time frame – for example, how long will it take you to come and review the patient? The nurses should also make suggestions concerning the treatment or intervention required. As this is the last communication in the assessment tool, expectations should be clarified on both sides.

Using the three prompts, raise the recommendation part of the SBAR.

An outline answer is provided below.

Answer

My recommendation concerning Mr Johnson is that I need you to come and review the patient. Can you please come to see the patient in the next (state how many minutes) or immediately. Is there anything I need to do in the meantime? – e.g. increase the oxygen? Request a portable chest X-ray, increase the frequency of the observations? By the time you get here, you would like me to (repeat what the receiver has said to you). For example, would you like me to get a chest X-ray organised?

SBAR is a simple and effective tool for communicating urgent and non-urgent patient assessment. It can be used in any clinical or non-clinical setting as it promotes patient safety and provides a structured format to communicate between nurses and other healthcare practitioners.

Chapter summary

The purpose of this chapter was to provide information on some of the most commonly used assessment tools in nursing. By understanding and gaining knowledge of these tools, student nurses should be able to develop skills that are pertinent to patient assessment. The list of tools is not exhaustive, but as a future graduate/registered nurse, the tools identified here should provide a foundation for understanding and performing patient assessment.

Activities: Brief outline answers

Activity 5.1   Critical thinking (p93)

See Figure 5.2 below for a fully labelled diagram.

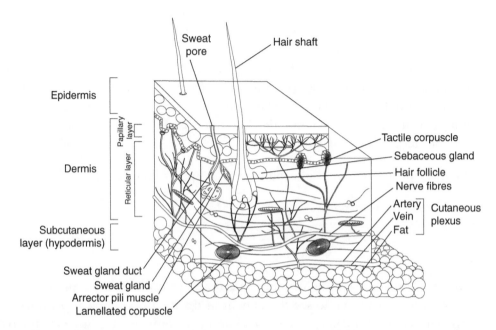

Figure 5.2   Accessory structures of the skin (Boore et al., 2016)

Activity 5.4   Critical thinking (p99)

Winston has scored a 2 and therefore is at high risk. Calvin should give dietary advice that can be used to maximise the patient's intake. He can do this by encouraging Winston to have small and frequent snacks. These should be high-energy and protein food and fluids. He can give the patient a food leaflet on how to maintain and prevent weight loss in hospital, or any similar advice material that is provided by the hospital. Calvin can also get oral nutritional supplements prescribed. He should also make a dietitian referral and commence a food and fluid intake chart (input/output).

The documents/forms Calvin needs to complete are: 1) a dietician referral form; 2) he should consider tissue viability referral; 3) commence a food chart; 4) commence a fluid balance chart; 5) he should update the patient's care plan; 6) he should review all these documents regularly and raise any concerns with the senior nurse on his shift.

After handing over to the nurses on the ward, Calvin can share his plan with the multidisciplinary team via the communication medium used. This may be a shared drive on the hospital computer or a communication book, or MDT meeting. If a patient board is used at the bedside, he can update some information there, remembering to maintain patient confidentiality.

Activity 5.5   Reflection (p101)

Example of initiatives and care plans you may have seen in place to prevent or reduce falls are listed below.

- The call bell is within reach of the patient to call for assistance.
- Patients are assessed for and wear safe footwear.

- Ensure that the bed is at the lowest level setting to the floor.
- Risk assessment for bedrails (if the patient attempts to climb over the bedrail, this will not be an appropriate measure).
- Fall alarm to alert staff when the patient is attempting to get up from the bed/chair unaided.
- Patients are assessed for and use the correct walking aid when mobilising.
- If the patient uses hearing aids and/or glasses, ensure they are used when mobilising.
- Refer the patient to the physiotherapist and/or occupational therapist if there is a need.
- Ensure that the patient's mobility plan is documented.
- Assess whether the patient needs additional staff to prevent a fall from occurring.
- Patients may be moved closer to the nurses' station so they can be observed.
- Ensure that the patient's medication is reviewed by the doctor and pharmacist.

Further reading

Edsberg, LE, Black, JM, Goldberg, M, McNichol, L, Moore, L and Sieggreen, M (2016) Revised National Pressure Ulcer Advisory Panel pressure injury staging system: revised pressure injury staging system. *Journal of Wound, Ostomy, and Continence Nursing, 43* (6): 585.

Useful websites

1. Use this website to gain a better understanding on how to complete a SSKIN assessment: **www.iow.nhs.uk/Downloads/SSKINBundle/SSKIN_Bundle_CompleteWeb.pdf**

2. To gain a quick overview of SSKIN, view this short video: **https://alpinehc.co.uk/blog/sskin-5-simple-steps-to-prevent-and-treat-pressure-ulcers/**

3. Use this website to learn how to assess the skin by the RCN: **https://rcni.com/hosted-content/rcn/first-steps/assessing-patients-skin**

4. Use this website for an explanation of AVPU: **www.youtube.com/watch?v=5FgsoAGyiJg**

5. Use this website to look at how to undertake a Waterlow assessment: **www.judy-waterlow.co.uk/waterlow_score.htm**

6. Use this website to read about falls prevention: **https://improvement.nhs.uk/resources/falls-prevention-resources/**

Chapter 6 Introduction to anatomy and physiology

Xabi Cathala and Alexandra Costa

NMC Standards of Proficiency for Registered Nurses

Platform 3: Assessing needs and planning care

Registered nurses prioritise the needs of people when assessing and reviewing their mental, physical, cognitive, behavioural, social and spiritual needs. They use information obtained during assessments to identify the priorities and requirements for person-centred and evidence-based nursing interventions and support. They work in partnership with people to develop person-centred care plans that take into account their circumstances, characteristics and preferences.

At the point of registration, the registered nurse will be able to:

3.2   demonstrate and apply knowledge of body systems and homeostasis, human anatomy and physiology, biology, genomics, pharmacology and social and behavioural sciences when undertaking full and accurate person-centred nursing assessments and developing appropriate care plans.

Platform 4: Providing and evaluating care

Registered nurses take the lead in providing evidence-based, compassionate and safe nursing interventions. They ensure that the care they provide and delegate is person-centred and of a consistently high standard. They support people of all ages in a range of care settings. They work in partnership with people, families and carers to evaluate whether care is effective and the goals of care have been met in line with their wishes, preferences and desired outcomes.

At the point of registration, the registered nurse will be able to:

4.5   demonstrate the knowledge and skills required to support people with commonly encountered physical health conditions, their medication usage and treatments, and act as a role model for others in providing high quality nursing interventions when meeting people's needs;

4.10 demonstrate the knowledge and ability to respond proactively and promptly to signs of deterioration or distress in mental, physical, cognitive and behavioural health and use this knowledge to make sound clinical decisions.

Chapter aims

After reading this chapter, you will be able to:

- understand the concept of homeostasis;
- develop knowledge and understanding of the functional anatomy and physiology of the respiratory system;
- have knowledge and understand the function of the circulatory system;
- have knowledge and understand the function of the renal system;
- have knowledge and understand the function of the central nervous system;
- have knowledge and understand the function of the gastrointestinal system;
- demonstrate an ability to apply function of the body to nursing assessment;
- be able to link an abnormal clinical assessment with a system's dysfunction.

Introduction

Nursing science comprises various topics – for example, psychology, sociology and biology. This chapter focuses on the anatomy and physiology of the human body, which includes the biological element of nursing science.

Anatomy and physiology is one of the cornerstones of nursing knowledge. Without sound knowledge of the body's anatomy and how it works (physiology), it will be difficult to provide the care needed for your patient. In this chapter, we look at the anatomy and physiology of the five most important human body systems: the respiratory system, the circulatory system, the renal system, the digestive system and central nervous system.

These systems are closely linked to each other to create the interesting functions of the human body. The chapter begins with explaining homeostasis and then takes you through the respiratory system, its anatomy and function. Here you learn about the different parts that make up the respiratory system – for example, the lungs and respiratory tract. The chapter helps you to understand the circulatory system, including how the heart works and how blood is transported across the body. The next sections cover the renal system, which is made up of the kidneys, and you will learn how they help to excrete toxins and produce urine. The chapter ends with the central nervous and digestive systems, where you will learn about how the nerves work to send messages to the body and also how to assess consciousness. In the final section on the digestive system, you will gain an understanding of how food is broken down and absorbed, and waste products excreted. The body manages all these functions by maintaining an equal balance of its internal system, known as homeostasis.

Homeostasis

To be able to perform fully without fault or distress, the body needs to maintain a constant internal environment. All systems keep a complex equilibrium to maintain the functioning of the body. All organs and tissues in the body have a specific role. Each function is linked with others to make a complex unity. They communicate with each other by neurotransmission, chemical reactions and hormones. You will learn later in the chapter – for example, in the section on the kidney system with the renin–angiotensin–aldosterone (RAA) pathway or the antidiuretic hormone (ADH) pathway – how the messages are sent and the reactions that occur to these messages. The overall working of this synchronisation is called 'homeostasis'. At all times, the body does everything it can do to maintain homeostasis. If the disturbance is too significant and all the mechanisms to maintain homeostasis fail, the person will become very ill and the knowledge and care of the healthcare worker will be necessary. Disease can present an acute onset or chronic pain can also disturb homeostasis. When we discuss the five major systems, we will remind you of the homeostatic mechanism.

The respiratory system

Let's start by looking at the respiratory system. We will use the case study and activity below to help you understand the anatomy and physiology of the respiratory system.

Case study: Mr Mabouthi

Mr Mabouthi is a 50-year-old East African patient on your ward. He rings the nurse call bell and when you arrive in the room, you find Mr Mabouthi breathless, cyanosed, fighting to catch his breath (referred to as dyspnoeic) and panicking. He is not able to complete full sentences before having to take a breath.

Activity 6.1 aims to identify how you understand the above case study, and how you may respond to such a situation.

Activity 6.1   Critical thinking

Answer the following questions:

- What is your understanding of the presentation of the patient's signs and symptoms?
- When you are faced with such a situation, what actions will you take?

An outline answer is provided at the end of the chapter.

Now that we have looked at the case study and Activity 6.1 above, we turn to the section on the anatomy of the respiratory system, which can help you to understand what was happening to Mr Mabouthi.

Anatomy of the respiratory system

The respiratory system is divided into three different parts: the airway (upper airway and lower airway), the lungs and the respiratory muscles (see Figure 6.1).

The airway – namely, the trachea and bronchi – deliver air from outside the lungs to the body. This includes the upper airway (the nose, mouth, pharynx, larynx) and the lower airway (the trachea, bronchi and bronchioles) (Marieb et al., 2018).

Activity 6.2 is designed to test your knowledge of the anatomy of the upper airway.

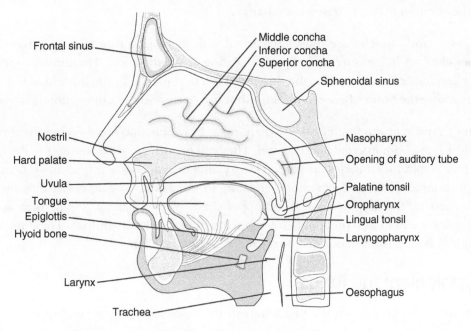

Figure 6.1   Upper respiratory tract (Boore et al., 2016)

Activity 6.2 Critical thinking

List the functions of the different parts of the upper airway in Figure 6.1.

An outline answer is provided at the end of the chapter.

Now that we have looked at the upper airway, we will turn our attention to the lower respiratory track where you will find the lungs.

Anatomy of the lungs

The lungs are soft cavities with the capacity to inflate and deflate. They are located in the intra-thoracic space above the diaphragm, protected by the ribcage (Marieb et al., 2018). There are two lungs – one on the right and one on the left. The main difference between the right and left lung is that the right lung has three lobes, whereas the left lung only has two. The left lung is smaller because it has to accommodate the heart, which is slightly orientated towards the left from the central position.

The circulatory network to the lungs is complex. For now, you need to understand that arteries and veins supply oxygenated blood to the body. One exception is that the pulmonary artery carries deoxygenated blood from the right side of the heart to the lungs, and the pulmonary vein carries oxygenated blood back to the left atrium of the heart.

The functional units of the lung are tiny sacs found at the end of the bronchioles, known as alveoli (Marieb et al., 2018). There are millions of these units in each lung, and they help to maintain gaseous exchange.

The respiratory muscles are those concerned with increasing thoracic capacity, which creates changes in pressure and allows inhalation and exhalation. The most important of the respiratory muscles is the diaphragm. It is a thin muscle at the bottom of the thorax, marking the border between the intrathoracic space and the intra-abdominal space.

Another muscle group that assists the diaphragm in its function are the intercostal muscles, which are both internal and external. They can be located between the ribs. Another group of respiratory muscles are the accessory muscles, which are inspiratory – i.e. they help with inhalation – and expiratory – relating to exhalation. The accessory muscles are located around the shoulders, neck and upper chest. When a patient is using their accessory muscles to help with breathing, it is often a sign of respiratory distress. These muscles help air to flow in (inhalation) and out (exhalation) of the lungs.

Physiology of the lungs

When we are talking about the physiology of the respiratory system, we are looking at the mechanism of breathing, which is also known as respiration. The mechanical function of the respiration process is to move air from outside the body to the inside, and the reverse from inside to outside of the body. The physiological function is to provide gaseous exchange between the blood and the alveoli. Let's have a look at a respiratory cycle.

Air enters the body through the nose via the nostril and nares. Passing through the nostril, the air is filtrated by tiny hairs, which clean the air of dust and other particles ready to enter the nasal cavity. The purpose of the nasal cavity, apart from conducting the air further down the respiratory track, is also to humidify the air – this is the process of making the air moist as it enters the respiratory tract. Once the air has been cleaned and humidified, it passes down to the pharynx and the larynx. The air now leaves the upper airway and makes its way to the lower airway via the trachea. The trachea is a rigid tube made of a ring of cartilage that you can feel at the bottom of the front of the neck.

The trachea is the only way that air can get into and out of the body. The trachea is divided into two – the right and the left bronchus. The right bronchus connects to the right lung and the left bronchus connects to the left lung. Finally, the air arrives in the alveoli through the bronchioles. At this stage, the transportation of the air into the lungs ends. Gaseous exchange then occurs in the alveoli (Marieb et al., 2018). The freshly inhaled air is highly concentrated in oxygen and passes into the bloodstream. The carbon dioxide contained in the bloodstream will be moved outside the body through exhalation and then pass into the air. The entrance of oxygen into the bloodstream and the exit of the carbon dioxide from the bloodstream is known as gas exchange. The air, which is now highly concentrated in carbon dioxide, will return to be released outside the body. This exchange is one of the mechanisms that maintain homeostasis (see Figure 6.2).

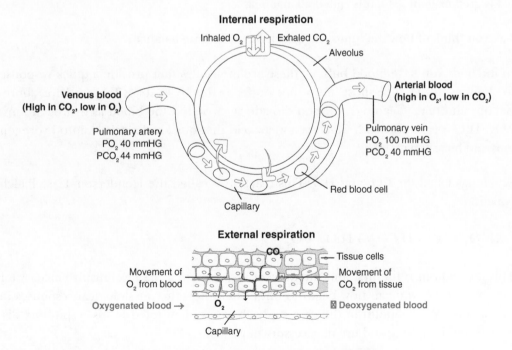

Figure 6.2 External and internal respiration (Boore et al., 2016)

The inspiratory muscles make inspiration possible – i.e. breathing in, or inhalation. The diaphragm and the external intercostal muscles contract. As a result, the intrathoracic volume increases, leading to the intrapulmonary pressure drop, allowing the air to enter. In exhalation – i.e. breathing out – the inspiratory muscles relax, the intrathoracic volume decreases and the intrapulmonary pressure rises. This action allows the air to exit from the lungs.

The pattern of the respiration is cyclic, with a respiratory rate of between 9 and 14 breaths per minute (Badriyah et al., 2014) and with an adequate lung expansion. An adequate expansion ensures that there is sufficient volume of air circulating in both lungs to oxygenate blood. You may hear this referred to as 'tidal volume'. For reference, an acceptable tidal volume is 500ml for a healthy adult or you can use the formula 7ml/kg.

Adequate oxygen concentration in the blood can be measured via the patient's oxygen saturations. An optimal gas exchange helps to maintain a constant internal environment known as homeostasis.

Apart from gaseous exchange, the lungs also help to maintain homeostasis by contributing to the acid base balance of the body. To maintain its function, the body needs to have a certain balance between acid and base. Acid is a substance that can provide an ion H+ and base is a substance that can accept an ion H+. As the quantity of ion H+, even in very acid solutions, is very small, a scale is used to measure it, known as the pH scale. The ideal pH for the body is 7.35–7.45. The pH can be measured in the blood, preferably in arterial blood. If the blood pH is below 7.35 it is called acidaemia; if the pH is greater than 7.45, it is called alkalaemia.

Can you think of how the lungs can affect the acid/ base balance?

In the body you have blood buffers, these are molecules that provide a quick response to changes in pH. The most important buffer is the HCO_3 (see Table 6.1 for abbreviations and their meaning). Carbon dioxide is carried in the blood as hydrogen ions. $CO_2 + H_2O$ = carbonic acid, which is a weak acid that quickly dissociates into hydrogen ions and bicarbonate ions.

The lungs expel the CO_2 and H_2O. This reaction is called the Henderson–Hasselbalch equation:

$$HCO_3^- + H^+ \rightarrow H_2CO_3 \rightarrow H_2O + CO_2$$

This mechanism is the first and the quicker response to a pH level disturbance. After careful reading, you can now begin to understand how the physiological responses in the patient, Mr Mabouthi in the case study above, is manifested in his respiratory distress (rapid breathing and use of accessory muscles).

Abbreviation	Meaning
RAA	Renin-angiotensin-aldosterone
ADH	Antidiuretic hormone
AV	Atrioventricular
ECG	Electrocardiogram
H_2O	Water
NaCl	Sodium chloride
HCO_3^-	Bicarbonate
H^+	Hydrogen
K^+	Potassium
ICF	Intracellular fluid
ECF	Extracellular fluid
$NaHCO_3^-$	Sodium bicarbonate

Table 6.1   Abbreviations and their meanings

Activity 6.3 is designed to help you reflect on your knowledge of the respiratory cycle. You can start by looking at what happens to your body when you inhale and exhale, or breathe in and out.

Activity 6.3   Reflection

In this activity, reflect on what physiological changes take place in a patient with breathing difficulties.

As this is a reflective exercise, no outline answer is provided.

From reflecting on Activity 6.3, you would have learned that the respiratory system is linked to the circulatory system.

The circulatory system

Anatomy of the circulatory system

When we talk about the circulatory system, people naturally think of the heart. The circulatory system is made up of much more than the heart itself. It includes all the vessels – veins, arteries and capillaries – and the heart.

The heart is located in the medial section of the thoracic cavity, between the two lungs (Marieb et al., 2018). The pointed part of the heart, called the apex, is directed towards the left. The heart is made up of muscle known as the myocardium, which is responsible for the contraction or beats of the heart.

The heart comprises four different chambers: the right atrium, right ventricle, left atrium and the left ventricle. As a student on a ward, you will hear colleagues talk about the right and left sides of the heart. The right side of the heart contains the right atrium and ventricle, which are separated from the left atrium and ventricle by a septum (Marieb et al., 2018). The right and left side of the heart initiate two different circuits with two completely different functions – the pulmonary circuit and the systemic circuit.

The pulmonary circuit

Venous blood enters the right atrium of the heart via the superior and inferior vena cavae. The right atrium is supplied by the superior and inferior vena cava. The right atrium communicates with the right ventricle through the right atrioventricular valve (tricuspid valve). The right ventricle pumps the blood straight into the pulmonary artery through the pulmonary semilunar valve. The blood then flows into the pulmonary circuit. After passing through the pulmonary capillaries (junction between arterioles and venules), the blood returns to the left atrium. The left ventricle communicates with the left atrium via the left atrioventricular valve (bicuspid valve). The left ventricle pumps the blood into the aorta through the aorta semilunar valve. The aorta is the largest artery in the human body.

At this point, the blood enters the systemic circuit. All the organs of the body will be perfused by oxygenated blood, and deoxygenated blood returns to the right side of the heart by the inferior and superior cava veins. The left ventricle is thicker than the right ventricle because of the stronger contraction needed to pump blood all around the body, while the right ventricle only has to pump blood to the lungs.

The blood passing through the heart does not nourish the myocardium. The blood supply that oxygenates and nourishes the myocardium is provided by the right and left coronary arteries. The base of the aorta is the origin of the coronary arteries, which supply blood to the myocardium. Any clots in one of these arteries result in an injury to the heart. This injury is called a myocardial infarction, commonly known as a heart attack.

We usually speak about arteries and veins as the main vessels in the cardiovascular circulatory system. There are three different types of vessels: the arteries, veins and capillaries. The arteries are the vessels that transport blood from the heart to the organs to deliver oxygen and nutrients. The veins are the vessels that return the blood from the organs to the heart. This blood is then poor in nutrients and oxygen. However, one exception exists: the pulmonary artery from the right ventricle to the lungs transports blood that is poor in oxygen and nutrients. In the same way, the pulmonary vein is the only vein in the human body carrying blood full of oxygen and nutrients.

The arteries and veins are connected to each other by the capillaries. The capillaries are tiny vessels that allow the exchange between arteries, veins and the organs. Their function is not the only difference between the arteries, veins and capillaries. Their structure is also different. The arteries and veins have three layers in their anatomy: the tunica intima (interior of the vessel), tunica media and tunica externa (exterior of the vessel).

The walls of the arteries are much thicker and stronger than walls of the veins. This allows the arteries to complete their function of carrying blood that is pressurised by the heart's contraction. Blood pressure in the veins is much lower, which explains why veins are thinner than arteries. As the veins are not under pressure, they use a valve system, closing and opening to create a flow to return the blood to the heart. This flow is mainly created by the contraction of the skeletal muscle. This explains why we encourage patients to keep moving as soon as possible after surgery to avoid complications.

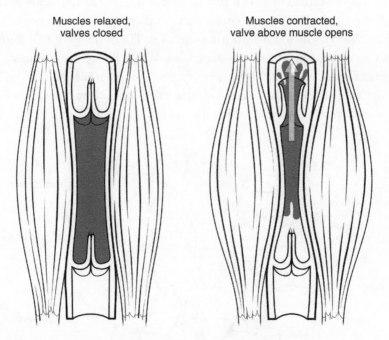

Figure 6.3 Blood flow in the lower leg (Boore et al., 2016)

The capillaries have only one layer – the tunica intima – which is one cell layer thick. This gives the capillaries the capacity to exchange blood with other organs in the body. The aim of the cardiovascular system is achieved by the smallest vessels (capillaries) of the body, keeping all the organs alive.

Physiology

The heart is the main pump of the body, which transports blood. The heart's function is to maintain a constant flow of blood through the body by contracting at around 60 to 90 times per minute. The function and contraction of the heart is automatic. A contraction is known as a heartbeat and is spontaneous.

To make this spontaneous contraction possible, an impulse is generated in the right atrium, which sends a signal to make the heart contract. This particular area is called the nodal note or sinoatrial node, and is responsible for the pacemaker function of the heart. Once the nodal system initiates depolarisation of the cells, this depolarisation will go through the muscle until the atrioventricular node catches the depolarisation. The atrioventricular (AV) node is responsible for spreading the electrical message from the nodal node to the ventricles by the atrioventricular bundle (known as the bundle of His); the bundle then branches into the Purkinje fibres. The conduction of the electrical message will result in a myocardial contraction. The atrioventricular node has an important role, acting as a conductor for the heart. The AV node is responsible for the conduction delay between the atrium and the ventricles. This delay is fundamental, allowing the ventricles to fill up with blood before their contraction. Without this delay, the heart would be inefficient. This electrical activity initiates the contraction of the heart as the message goes through the heart. The atrium contracts first, the right atrioventricular valve opens and allows the blood to flow down to the ventricles. Then, the AV node, after receiving the electrical message, sends it to the ventricles. While the electrical message is going through the ventricles, the blood fills them up and the atrioventricular valve closes. The ventricles then contract and the two semilunar valves open into the pulmonary vein or the aorta. This completes the cycle, which then starts again (see Figure 6.4).

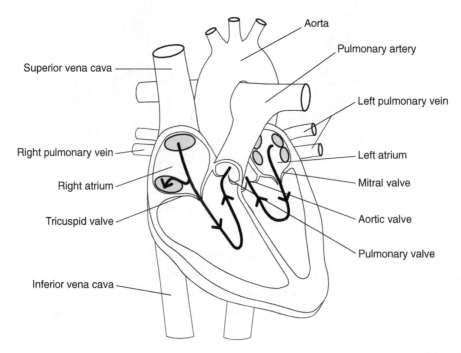

Figure 6.4 Blood flow and contraction of the heart (Boore et al., 2016)

This electrical message spreads through the heart from the nodal node and creates what we call a rhythm and pulse. The rhythm has to be regular and between 51 to 90 beats per minute to be recognised as normal or sinus rhythm. This can be felt as a pulse or heartbeat.

In Activity 6.4, you need to work with a colleague to practise how to feel for and check for a pulse rate.

Activity 6.4   Teamworking

Find one of your student peers and practise finding their pulse.

- Record the number of beats.
- Describe what you feel when checking for the pulse.

As a nurse, you will feel for the amplitude – whether it is weak or full/ bounding – rate and regularity.

As this is a teamwork exercise, no outline answers are provided. Discuss and record your findings with your colleague at the end of the activity.

As the heart rhythm is an electrical message, it can be recorded by an electrocardio-gram (ECG). This record can be printed off as a trace and analysed by a competent healthcare worker to identify any abnormalities. This rhythm has a definite pattern. It must have a P wave, a QRS wave and a T wave. Where the P wave is related to the atrium contraction, the QRS wave is the ventricular contraction and the T wave is the relaxation of the ventricle. The relaxation of the atrium is hidden by the QRS wave. If it is regular (between 60 to 90 beats per minute), it is called a sinus rhythm, and each QRS wave has a P wave beforehand (see Figure 6.5).

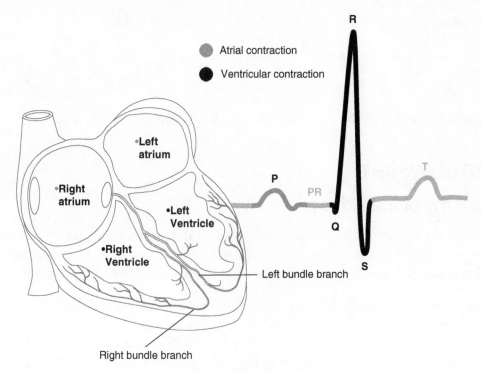

Figure 6.5   A normal sinus rhythm showing QRS complex (Boore et al., 2016)

The sinus rhythm is the normal pattern of the heart rhythm. If the ECG is different from this pattern, it is abnormal, and the cause of this abnormality needs to be investigated. Abnormalities are called arrhythmias.

The case study below looks at how someone with a cardiac problem may present at hospital.

Case study: Mr Simmonds

Mr Simmonds is 60 years old and walks into the A&E Department. He complains of a chest pain and is feeling dizzy. You can see that he is starting to become short of breath. You can also see that he looks pale and sweaty. He is overweight for his height.

In Activity 6.5, you will need to look at how you identify the care that will be needed, using your knowledge of the cardiovascular system.

Activity 6.5   Critical thinking

For this activity, you will need to make a list.

* What is your understanding of Mr Simmonds's presentation in the A&E Department?
* Based on your understanding, what actions will you undertake?

An outline answer is provided at the end of the chapter.

The next section focuses on the renal system, and its anatomy and function.

Renal system

Anatomy of the kidneys

Although the kidneys are well known as the organs that makes urine, their function is much more than that. By the end of the chapter, you will understand why the kidneys are important and why they are one of the first organs we look at in the ill patient.

There are two kidneys in the human body, although one kidney is sufficient to achieve its function and maintain homeostasis. Try to identify where your kidneys are inside your body. Most people will locate the kidneys in the lower part of the back, which is not entirely correct. The kidneys are in the lower posterior part of the rib cage. The bony structure of the rib cage acts as a protective shield to the kidneys (see Figure 6.6).

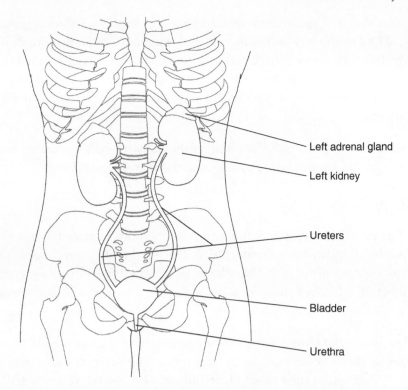

Figure 6.6 Position of the kidneys in the rib cage (Boore et al., 2016)

The kidneys are relatively small organs, around 12cm (5in) long and 6cm (2½in) wide. The shape of the kidney is often compared to a kidney bean. The right kidney is lower than the left due to the position of the liver. The functional unit of the kidney is called the nephron. There are over one million nephrons in each kidney. The nephron is made up of the renal corpuscle and the renal tubule. The network of capillaries in the corpuscle is called the glomerulus, which is surrounded by a structure called the Bowman's capsule. The renal tubule is made up of the proximal, intermediate (referred to as the Loop of Henle) and distal tubule. The main function of the nephron is to regulate water and soluble substances through filtering blood. (See Useful websites at the end of the chapter, link no. 5, for further information on nephrons.) From the kidneys, there are two slender tubes about 30cm (12in) each and 6mm in diameter called ureters. Each ureter runs and is connected from the kidney to the bladder.

The urinary bladder is a smooth muscular sac that is expandable and stores urine temporarily. The bladder wall contains three layers of smooth muscle. An empty bladder is about 5–7.5cm (2–3in) in length. As the urine accumulates, the volume of the bladder increases. A bladder about 12.5cm (5in) long is usually full and will hold approximately 500ml of urine. The kidneys produce urine continuously. The function of the bladder is to store urine until it is released.

The urethra is the tube that carries the urine from the bladder to outside the body. Between the urethra and the bladder there are two sphincters: an internal urethral sphincter (involuntary sphincter) and an external urethra sphincter (voluntarily controlled). The urethra is different in men and women. In men, the length is approximately 20cm (8in). In women, the urethra is much shorter, about 3–4cm (1½in). The fact that a woman's urethra is short means that there is a higher risk of bladder infection. In men, the urethra forms part of the reproductive system and allows the exit of urine and semen.

It is essential to have a good understanding of the anatomy of the renal system because it will allow you to understand the physiology and diseases of the system.

Physiology

The main function of the kidney is the filtration of blood, to clear the bloodstream of the waste produced by the body (Peate, 2016). During the filtration process, the kidney produces and excretes urine to the bladder to be removed from the body. For the renal system to function effectively, it needs a blood supply, a kidney, a ureter, a bladder and a urethra.

The blood supply to the kidney arrives via the renal artery. This artery will be the origin to numerous smaller arteries such as the arterioles. The arterioles are the vessels that will assist with filtration in the kidney. Once filtration is finished, venous circulation will return the blood to the inferior vena cava.

Nephrons are responsible for blood filtration. Filtration and urine formation is accomplished in three processes: the glomerular filtration, the tubular reabsorption and the tubular secretion. Each process needs to be completed to ensure an adequate kidney function and to maintain homeostasis.

The glomerular filtration is the first step of the process and occurs in the glomerular capsule. This capsule consists of the glomerular capillaries from the afferent arteriole. When blood first enters here, glomerular filtration occurs.

The solutes smaller than proteins (including urea, creatinine and uric acid) and water are removed from the capillaries of the glomerular capsule and passed into the renal tubule based on the pressure in blood vessels. Water (H_2O), sodium chloride (NaCl), bicarbonate (HCO_3^-), hydrogen (H+), urea, glucose, amino acids and some drugs will be removed from the bloodstream to the renal tube.

The three parts of the renal tube – the proximal tubule, Loop of Henle, distal tubule – come into function. In the proximal tubule, the main reabsorption process occurs. The NaCl, HCO_3^-, glucose and amino acids are actively transported from the renal tubule to the capillaries. Water is passively transported from the renal tubule to the capillaries. The tubular secretion process also occurs in the proximal tubule; some drugs, poisons and H+ will be actively transported from the capillaries to the renal tubule. In the second part of the renal tubule (nephron loop), only the reabsorption process occurs. Here, water will be passively moved from the nephron loop to the capillaries. The NaCl will be moved from the nephron loop to the capillaries. In the last part of the renal tubule (distal tubule), the NaCl is actively removed from the distal tubule to the capillaries. Some active secretion of potassium (K+) and drugs from the capillaries to the distal tubule will occur. The liquid will then enter in the collecting duct where again NaCl will be actively transported, H_2O and urea will be removed from the collecting duct to the capillaries. K+ will be secreted from the capillaries to the collecting duct. Then urine is drained into the ureter to be stored in the bladder until elimination.

Through the filtration process, the kidneys make urine and remove the waste products from the body. It is not the only function, because during filtration the electrolytes (NaCl, K+), bicarbonate, amino acids, hydrogen, glucose and water exchange regulate their concentration in the bloodstream. The regulation of those molecules will have an impact on each system of the body in a different way. For example, the electrolytes and water have an impact on the cardiovascular system, and the regulation of hydrogen and bicarbonate have an impact on the respiratory system. That explains the central part of the kidneys in maintaining the body's constant internal environment (homeostasis). It is essential that a normal renal function is maintained.

The main component in the human body is water; in terms of body weight, it constitutes around 50 per cent in women and 60 per cent in men (Marieb et al., 2018). This water occupies a different location in the body, known as compartments. The main compartment is the intracellular fluid (ICF), the second is the interstitial fluid (ECF) and the third is plasma. The interstitial fluid and plasma are known as extracellular fluid (ECF). The plasma – part of the blood – is the main conduit connecting the organs of the body. In the body, the water's exchange occurs continuously. Three main systems are used in the water regulation – the respiratory, gastrointestinal and renal systems. The system mainly responsible for water regulation is the renal system. To achieve this function, the kidneys use two different mechanisms requiring hormones and enzymes (a substance produced by a living organism that acts as a catalyst to bring about a specific biochemical reaction: the renin–angiotensin–aldosterone pathway (RAA) and the antidiuretic hormone pathway (ADH)).

The RAA pathway takes place at the entrance of the glomerular capsule. A decrease in the renal arterial pressure will be detected by the juxtaglomerular apparatus (group of cells in contact with the afferent arteriole and efferent arteriole). This low pressure in the arteriole stimulates the juxtaglomerular cells to secrete an enzyme called renin. In the presence of renin enzyme, angiotensinogen is converted into angiotensin I, angiotensin II. This conversion is aided by ACE (angiotensin converting enzymes), which are found in the lungs. An arterial vasoconstriction, an increase filtration pressure and a stimulation of the adrenal cortex are conducted by angiotensin II. The adrenal cortex is a structure located in the adrenal gland at the top of the kidney. Angiotensin II stimulates the release of the hormone aldosterone from the adrenal glands. This increases the reabsorption of Na^+ in the Loop of Henle, which in turn increases the reabsorption of water, resulting from an increase in sodium chloride reabsorption from distal tubules and collecting ducts. As the water has the same pathway as sodium chloride, it is reabsorbed simultaneously with sodium chloride, which results in an increase in blood volume and blood pressure. For each unit or milliosmoles of sodium chloride reabsorbed, one unit or milliosmole of potassium is secreted into the renal tubule. This mechanism then acts on water regulation and the electrolyte balance.

The second mechanism is the ADH (anti-diuretic hormone) pathway, which begins by the stimulation of the pituitary gland (part of the brain) by an increase of the blood osmolarity. The ADH released increases the permeability of the distal and conducting tubules in the nephron, resulting in the water being reabsorbed into the bloodstream. The water concentration in the blood increases and the osmolarity decreases. This change of osmolarity inhibits the ADH secretion. This second mechanism acts on the water balance of the human body.

Another function of the kidneys is to maintain the body's acid balance. This is achieved by working together with the respiratory system. The kidneys have buffers known as bicarbonate (HCO_3^-) and hydrogen ($H+$) and they help to maintain the acid balance (pH) in the blood. A low blood pH stimulates the tubular cells to secrete $H+$ into the filtrate. The cells then remove acid from the blood. To maintain the balance, $NA+$ is diffused from the filtrate to the blood.

In this process, $NA+$ is combined with bicarbonate (HCO_3^-) to form sodium bicarbonate ($NAHCO_3^-$), which is secreted into the blood. Through this reaction, the pH is corrected from a (low or high) acid to normal range. You can see when this reaction occurs on a blood gas test by a rising HCO_3^- and a corrected pH. This reaction can happen the other way around if the blood pH is high. This acid/base regulation by the kidney is not the first process, however. The first and quicker way to correct this acid balance disturbance is by the respiratory system described at the beginning of the chapter.

The respiratory system helps to maintain the balance of acids and bases in the body by controlling the blood levels of carbonic acid. CO_2 (carbon dioxide) in the blood reacts with H_2O to form carbonic acid. The levels of these two (CO_2 and carbonic acid) are in equilibrium in the blood, where homeostasis is maintained. When the level of CO_2 in the blood rises, the excess CO_2 reacts with water to form extra carbonic acid; the effects of this are that blood pH is lowered. The respiratory system addresses this by getting the body to increase the rate and/or depth of breathing. The main aim of this action is to allow greater exhalation of CO_2. This loss or reduction of CO_2 from the body lowers the levels of carbonic acid in blood, thus correcting the pH (upwards), bringing it to normal levels. Rapid deep breathing – for example, hyperventilation – removes CO_2 in the blood, which reduces the level of carbonic acid, making the blood too alkaline. The correction process works in the opposite direction to low acid (pH) (discussed earlier) to maintain normal range.

When the respiratory system is not strong enough to correct pH levels or fails to do so, the kidney acid/base regulation will take over this role.

Urine production is an important function of the renal system and well-functioning kidneys can produce good quality urine, while those affected can produce poor quality.

As a nurse, you will need to assess a patient's urine to identify the differences in urine quality. As we conclude this section, think of what you will look for when assessing a patient's urine.

In this chapter so far, we have covered the respiratory, circulatory and renal systems. In the case study below, we bring all three systems together so you can see how they work in clinical presentations.

Case study: Mrs Johti

Mrs Johti is 50 years old from a Pakistani background. She was admitted for observations because she was feeling generally unwell. Her heart rate is 68 and irregular, her blood pressure is 102/49. Her respiratory rate is 29 breaths per minute and on room air, her oxygen saturations are 89 per cent. You observe that she is in a negative fluid balance in that she appears to have excreted 1,000ml of fluid more than she has ingested.

Activity 6.6   Critical thinking

After reading the case study above, think and map out how the three systems are connected.

As this activity is for your own research, no outline answer is provided.

Central nervous system

We will now have a simple and broad approach to the neurological system. Before starting with the theory, read the following case study and reflect on Activity 6.7.

Case study: Mr Luis

Mr Luis is a patient originally from Spain on an orthopaedics ward recovering from a fractured femur, for which he has had surgery. On assessment, you observe that Mr Luis is awake, confused, but able to speak in full sentences. He has good upper motor power, but he is unable to lift his legs, wiggle/move his toes or bend his knees. He reports no sensation when you touch his legs. You notice that he has an epidural made up of bupivaccine 0.125 per cent and 4mcg of fentanyl per ml in progress running at 6ml/hr.

Activity 6.7   Critical thinking

Based on the assessment you have just performed:

1. What do you think is happening with Mr Luis?

2. What nursing interventions will you carry out?

3. Using the link for the Glasgow Coma Scale (GCS) (see Useful websites at the end of the chapter, link no. 6), calculate Mr Luis's score.

An outline answer is provided at the end of the chapter.

Now that you know how to perform a GCS assessment, identify reasons for motor responses and consider nursing intervention, we will now look at the brain and central nervous system.

The nervous system

The brain, spinal cord and nerves comprise the nervous system. Together, these structures control all the body's functions and coordinate how the body's organs work. We can divide the neurological system into the central nervous system (CNS) and the peripheral nervous system (PNS) (Porth, 2011).

The CNS – brain, brain stem and spinal cord – is situated within the skull and vertebral column. Immediately below these bony structures we find the meninges – pia mater, arachnoid and dura mater – that protect the CNS.

Figure 6.7 shows the direct motor pathway of the central nervous system.

The cerebrum is divided into two parts or hemispheres. They are joined by the corpus callosum. The cerebral cortex is divided into four lobes: frontal, parietal, temporal and occipital. The function of the cerebrum is to recognise the sensory input, process this information and then generate an adequate response (Adam and Osborne, 2005).

The spinal cord is located in the upper two-thirds of the canal of the vertebral column; its nerves emerge through the vertebral column and form branches that gradually grow smaller until they reach the skin and muscles. There are 32 pairs of spinal nerves: 8 cervical, 12 thoracic, 5 lumbar, 5 sacral and 2 coccygeal (Porth, 2011). These nerves establish the communication from their correspondent body segments through the afferent neurons to the CNS, where the information will be processed and then the efferent neurons carry information from the CNS to the effector organs (Porth, 2011).

The brain stem is formed by the midbrain, pons varolii and medulla oblongata, and links the brain to the spinal cord. It is located on the posterior part of the cranium and the

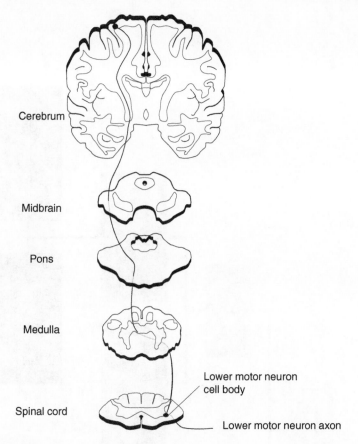

Cerebrum

Midbrain

Pons

Medulla

Lower motor neuron
cell body

Spinal cord

Lower motor neuron axon

Figure 6.7   Direct pathway of the central nervous system (Boore et al., 2016)

majority of cranial nerves originate in the brainstem (Adam and Osborne, 2005). If a person sustains any injury at this level of the CNS, the consequences can be life altering.

The cerebellum is responsible for fine dexterity and movements, and also for the balance of the body, by influencing the motor systems, as well as maintenance of a stable posture.

A protective and supportive fluid for the brain and spinal cord, called the cerebrospinal fluid (CSF), lies under the arachnoid meninges in the subarachnoid space (Porth, 2011). It is clear in appearance/colour. It should not contain any blood; if blood is present, then your patient is very ill. It is common for doctors to take a sample of CSF to diagnose some neurological diseases and infections. This procedure is called a lumbar puncture. In the activity below, consider why a lumbar puncture will be undertaken.

Activity 6.8   Critical thinking

Give three reasons why a lumbar puncture will be performed.

An outline answer is provided at the end of the chapter.

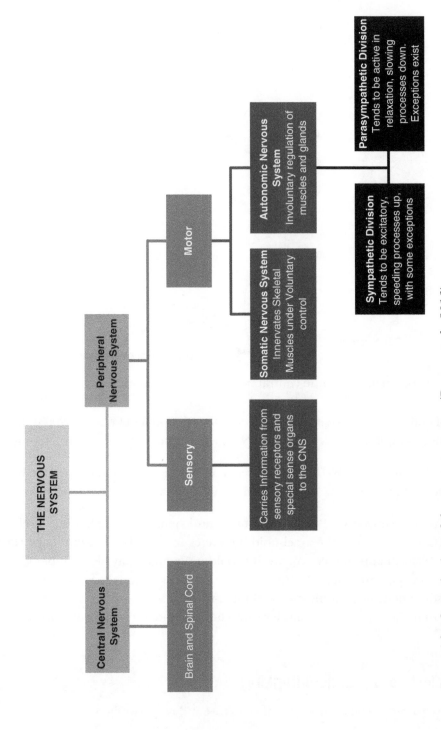

Figure 6.8 Organisation of the nervous system (Boore et al., 2016)

Now that you are beginning to understand the central nervous system, the focus of the next section is on the peripheral nervous system (PNS). Figure 6.8 shows you how the central and peripheral nervous systems are organised.

The PNS includes all the neural structures outside the skull and vertebral column.

Physiology

There are two types of nerve cells in the nervous tissue: neurons and supporting cells.

Neurons communicate with each other through structures called synapses in presence of neurotransmitters (Adam and Osborne, 2005). The synapses can be electrical or chemical (excitatory and inhibitory). Electrical synapses allow the movement of ions through gap junctions that work as bridges between the neurons. Chemical synapses comprise the production of a neurotransmitter or neuromodulator by the neuron's membranes that will fill in a gap between the neurons known as synaptic cleft (Porth, 2011). The most common neurotransmitters in the synapses are acetylcholine, noradrenaline and dopamine (see Figure 6.9).

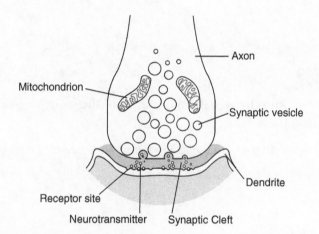

Figure 6.9   A synapse (Boore et al., 2016)

There are different types of supporting cells: in the PNS there are the Schwann and satellite cells and in the CNS the oligodendrocytes, astrocytes, microglial cells and ependymal cells. Their main role is to protect and give metabolic support to the neurons, allowing for normal neural function.

Before we look at the metabolic needs of the nervous system, we will explain metabolism.

Metabolism is the term used to describe the chemical reactions that take place in order to maintain the living status in the body's cells. Metabolism also helps with the removal of nitrogenous wastes from the body and uses the conversion of food into building blocks such as proteins, lipids, some carbohydrates and nucleic acids.

The brain represents 2 per cent of the body's weight, which might lead to a misconception of low metabolic needs. In fact, it receives about 15 per cent of the resting cardiac output and requires a continuous supply of glucose and oxygen, consuming 80 per cent of the total body oxygen. If a decrease of oxygen supply occurs, the patient will present with confusion and loss of consciousness, and if that progresses, the patient will go into cardiac arrest and neural cell death will occur.

In summary, the neurological system is a complex structure that controls all body functions, depends on oxygen and glucose input, and also on homeostasis to function appropriately. In the next section, the gastrointestinal system is presented.

Gastrointestinal system

This section starts with an activity that is designed to test your knowledge of the gastrointestinal system and its various parts.

Activity 6.9

With your own knowledge, schematically draw the gastrointestinal system and label the main parts.

For a fully labelled diagram of the digestive system, see Figure 6.11 on page 136.

Anatomy

The gastrointestinal (GI) tract is a long system that allows our body to ingest and digest food while absorbing nutrients from them. This process involves several organs working together. A simple way to understand and visualise the GI tract and its anatomy is to think of a hollow tube surrounded by a wall made up of five layers: the inner layer is called the mucosa layer, which produces mucous and protects the canal; second is the submucosal layer, which is made up of connective tissue and holds the blood vessels, nerves and structures that secret digestive enzymes; the third and fourth layers are the circular and longitudinal muscular layers, which are responsible for the movement of the gut content; the fifth layer is the outer layer and is called the peritoneum, a serous membrane that supports the bowel (see Figure 6.10).

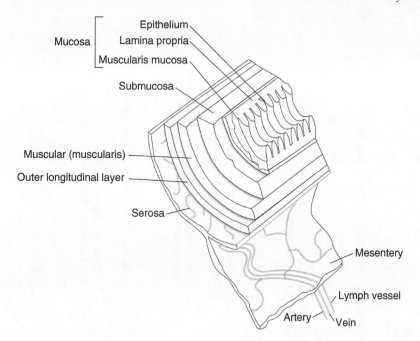

Figure 6.10   A tubular structure of the gastrointestinal tract (Boore et al., 2016)

Starting from the top, the mouth is the entry for food into the GI tract and the anus is the exit of the residual products after digestion and absorption. The GI tract is divided into the upper GI tract: the oesophagus and stomach; and the middle GI tract: the duodenum, jejunum and ileum. All of these parts together form the small intestine. The lower GI tract comprises the cecum, colon, rectum and the anal canal; together they form the large intestine (see Figure 6.11).

The GI tract also has some accessory organs: the salivary glands, liver, gall bladder and pancreas.

Physiology

Now that you have attempted to draw the GI tract and read a bit more on its structure, let us look at the physiology of the GI. As we ingest food, the salivary glands produce saliva. The saliva protects the oral mucosa, coats the food, making it easy to move, and has an antimicrobial action that cleans the mouth and initiates digestion because it contains ptyalin, a type of amylase. This enzyme helps in the breakdown of starch that is present in food into maltose and dextrin, which can then be absorbed into the GI system. It is important to note that the breakdown of starch is only started in the mouth and is completed in the ileum.

The oesophagus, also known as the gullet, is about 25cm (10in) in length and is a muscular tube that connects the mouth to the stomach. The oesophagus starts and ends

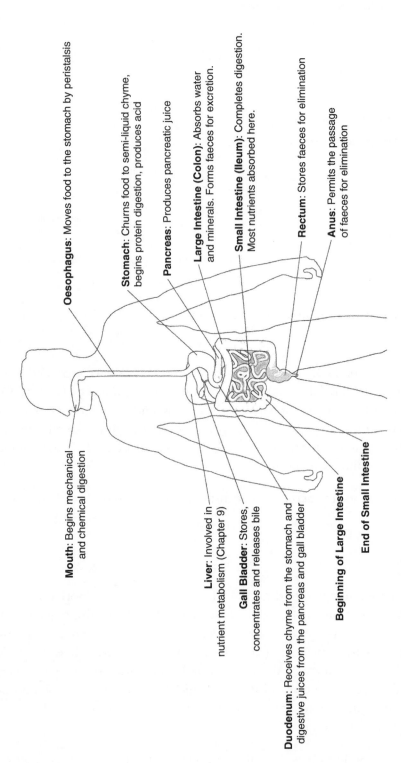

Figure 6.11   The gastrointestinal tract and accessory organs (Boore et al., 2016)

Oesophagus: Moves food to the stomach by peristalsis

Stomach: Churns food to semi-liquid chyme, begins protein digestion, produces acid

Pancreas: Produces pancreatic juice

Large Intestine (Colon): Absorbs water and minerals. Forms faeces for excretion.

Small Intestine (Ileum): Completes digestion. Most nutrients absorbed here.

Rectum: Stores faeces for elimination

Anus: Permits the passage of faeces for elimination

Mouth: Begins mechanical and chemical digestion

Liver: Involved in nutrient metabolism (Chapter 9)

Gall Bladder: Stores, concentrates and releases bile

Duodenum: Receives chyme from the stomach and digestive juices from the pancreas and gall bladder

Beginning of Large Intestine

End of Small Intestine

with a sphincter, the main purpose of which is to control the entry of food and liquids, and also to avoid reflux of food from the stomach. Once chewing begins, the food, together with saliva, forms a bolus and, with the help of the tongue, is passed to the oesophagus. As you swallow the bolus, the wall of the oesophagus contracts and pushes the food down to the stomach using this contractual method. This action is known as peristalsis.

The stomach (Figure 6.12) is a pear-shaped structure about 25cm (10in) long; it has the capacity to expand to a litre with food contents. The stomach sits in the upper part of the abdomen, below the lower oesophageal sphincter. It links the oesophagus to the small intestine. The stomach is a highly acidic environment and, together with the peristaltic movements, it promotes digestion. The gastric acid secretion depends on gastrin and acetylcholine. It has a diurnal rhythm and can be affected by smell, taste, chewing, swallowing, ingestion of alcohol or caffeine, glucose levels, distension of the stomach wall and digested proteins in the bowel (see Figure 6.12).

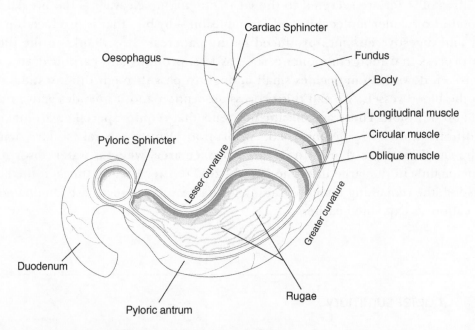

Figure 6.12 Parts of the stomach (Boore et al., 2016)

After leaving the stomach, the material/food, now called chyme, reaches the small intestine. The upper part of the small intestine is the duodenum, followed by the jejunum and the lower part is the ileum. At this level, the chyme undergoes different processes that will allow further digestion, absorption and movement to the large intestine. The pancreas, gall bladder and liver are close to the stomach. They produce juices and enzymes (chemicals) that help digestion. The duodenum is connected to the common bile duct and the pancreatic duct. The bile produced in the liver and stored in the gallbladder is released into the duodenum through the common bile duct. The pancreatic duct allows the digestive enzymes produced by the pancreas to pass to the duodenum. These enzymes are secreted in an inactivated form and become active once in the small intestine (Porth, 2011).

The lower GI tract, also known as the large intestine, is formed, as mentioned before, of the cecum, colon, rectum and anus. The cecum connects the small intestine to the colon (ascending, transverse and descending), the main functions of the colon include: absorption of water, folic acid, ammonia and electrolytes; mucus secretion, and lastly movement of the contents to the rectum. The rectum fills occasionally and, if appropriate, defecation will occur through the anus (Porth, 2011).

Digestion, absorption and waste products

Digestion takes place mainly in the small intestine, even though for carbohydrates and proteins this process starts in the stomach. It includes hydrolysis – every day 7–8 litres of water are secreted to the GI tract; enzyme cleavage – the breakdown of food into smaller molecules; and fat emulsion – by bile that is produced in the liver and digestive enzymes produced by the pancreas. It is thanks to the digestion process that food components such as fats, proteins and carbohydrates can be broken down into molecules small enough to pass through the intestinal wall into the blood vessels. We call this process absorption and it includes active transport and diffusion. There are specific nutrients that require special environmental conditions in order to be absorbed. Absorption of nutrients takes place mainly in the small intestine thanks to its large surface area, whereas water absorption occurs mainly in the large intestine (Porth, 2011). After passing through the large intestine, the remaining materials, also known as waste products, are eliminated by defecation, as explained earlier.

Chapter summary

In this chapter, we aimed to link the NMC domain nursing practice and decision-making related competencies to anatomy and physiology. It is important that as a student nurse you develop your knowledge and understanding of the main body systems – namely, the respiratory, cardiac, renal, nervous and gastrointestinal systems. The ability to recognise how these systems work to produce a balanced body – i.e. homeostasis – will help you to identify when dysfunction occurs and what you may need to do to support the organs and their systems to recover. We have recommended some useful electronic resources for you to use to further develop your knowledge and understanding.

Activities: Brief outline answers

Activity 6.1   Critical thinking (p115)

The initial understanding is that the patient is in respiratory distress, which is often characterised by one or more of the signs that the patient is exhibiting – i.e. breathlessness, cyanosed, dyspnoeic, panicking to breathe and unable to complete full sentences before having to take a breath.

You will need to assess your patient's airway and breathing. With regard to their airway, is the patient able to respond in full sentences? If not, are there any airway blockages or adjuncts that may be preventing them from replying to you in full sentences? After confirming airway patency, you will need to assess the patient's breathing. You should check their respiratory rate and depth, and look at the rise of their chest expansion – is it equal and symmetrical? Check the patient's oxygen saturation and whether they are on any supplemental oxygen.

Oxygen should be prescribed, but in an emergency situation you can give 15 litres via a rebreathe mask.

If you are unsure what to do, you should call for help from your mentor or a member of the team.

Activity 6.2   Critical thinking (p116)

The upper airway is made up of the following:

The nasal cavity The function of the nasal cavity is to allow air to enter the respiratory system through inhalation. The nasal cavity warms, moisturises and filters air before it enters the lungs.

The nasopharynx The function of the nasopharynx is to allow the person to breathe through their nose. It allows the movement of air from the nose and mouth to the larynx.

The oropharynx The oropharynx allows air to move to and from the nasal cavity. A flap made up of connective tissue called the epiglottis is located at the bottom of the oropharynx and serves as a guide to ensure that food does not enter the respiratory system.

The larynx The larynx connects the pharynx to the trachea (windpipe) and its function is to allow air to safely pass through it by not allowing food, drink and other foreign particles to block the airway and enter the lower respiratory track.

The laryngopharynx It is part of the pharynx and connects the mouth and nasal cavities to the oesophagus. It ensures that air is moved to the trachea and food to the oesophagus; through its function it ensures that each goes to the correct location.

Activity 6.5   Critical thinking (p124)

This is based on your understanding of the cardiovascular system. You will be correct in thinking that there is a problem with Mr Simmonds's cardiovascular system. You may want to link his chest pain and dizzy feelings to low blood pressure. Your understanding of his shortness of breath can be further informed by your knowledge of the respiratory system and its connection to the cardiovascular system. Can you think why he may have a change of colour and become sweaty?

- Read link no. 3 in the Useful websites section at the end of the chapter.
- You will want to assess his circulation and breathing, as these two appear to be affected.
- To assess circulation, check his pulse. You may want to recall Activity 6.5.

- You should also check his blood pressure and record this and his pulse rate.
- You should assess his breathing as described in Activity 6.1. Based on your recorded observation, you may have to administer oxygen.
- Other actions to consider are to do a full blood screen, an arterial blood gas and an ECG to confirm his heart rhythm.

If you feel unsure of the correct actions, seek help from a senior clinician or your mentor.

Activity 6.7   Critical thinking (p130)

There may be several reasons for Mr Luis's confusion – for example, he could be hypoxic or having post-surgery confusion, or his opioid medication could be contributing to his confusion. For his lower limbs motor responses, this can be due to the epidural. Go to link no. 7 in Useful websites at the end of the chapter to learn more about epidurals and how to assess dermatones.

- The first thing you can do is to ensure that your patient is safe.
- Perform an A–E assessment – this will help you to determine his respiratory status, which can be contributing to his confusion. Report the results to your mentor.
- You will want to perform a GCS and report the results to your mentor.
- You will want to consider the effect of the epidural and discuss it with your mentor. Your mentor may suggest reducing the rate of the epidural.
- Using the link for the Glasgow Coma Scale (Useful websites, link no. 6), calculate Mr Luis's score:
- Based on the Glasgow Coma Scale, the patient is scoring 9/15.
- Eyes opening = 4
- Verbal response = 4
- Best motor response = 1

Activity 6.8   Critical thinking (p131)

1. To gain a diagnosis of illness – for example, meningitis, encephalitis or certain cancers involving the brain and spinal cord.

2. To determine if there is bleeding in the brain, particularly in the subarachnoid space.

3. To remove some fluid to reduce the pressure in the brain or spine.

Further reading

Boore, J, Cook, N and Shepherd, A (2016) *Essentials of Anatomy and Physiology for Nursing Practice.* London: SAGE.

This is an essential read if you want to gain further knowledge on the five systems discussed in this chapter.

Peate, I and Nair, M (2015) *Anatomy and Physiology for Nurses at a Glance.* John Wiley & Sons.

Parts 4 and 5 are recommended reading for the respiratory system and gastrointestinal tract.

Thomas, N (ed.) (2008) *Renal Nursing.* Elsevier Health Sciences.

This text is written by a professor of real nursing. If you want to understand and learn about dialysis, it is a recommended text.

Watson, R (2011) *Anatomy and Physiology for Nurses E-Book.* Elsevier Health Sciences.

This text is written by a professor of nursing. The following three chapters are recommended for further reading: Control and Coordination; Internal Transport; Nutrition and Elimination.

Useful websites

1. Use this website to gain a better understanding of the respiratory system: **www.youtube. com/watch?v=kacMYexDgHg&frags=pl%2Cwn**

2. Use this website to gain a better understanding of the cardiac cycle: **www.youtube.com/ watch?v=IS9TD9fHFv0**

3. Use this website to get a better understanding of acute coronary syndrome: **www.youtube. com/watch?v=TBG9Jw3yd9I**

4. Use this website for a visual image of the kidney: **https://radiologykey.com/wp-content/ uploads/2016/03/c00091_f091-004-9780702042959.jpg**

5. Use this website to gain a better understanding of the structure of nephrons and their functions: **www.youtube.com/watch?v=QsSdAXv5BEM&frags=pl%2Cwn**

6. Use this website to complete Activity 6.7 on calculating the Glasgow Coma Scale: **www. glasgowcomascale.org/**

7. Use this website to gain a better understanding of assessing dermatones: **www.youtube.com/ watch?v=wsB2IaOojdc**

8. Use this website for a better understanding of the central nervous system: **www.youtube. com/watch?v=44B0ms3XPKU**

9. Use this website to gain a better understanding of the digestive system: **www.youtube.com/ watch?v=_QYwscALNng**

Chapter 7 Person-centred care

From secondary to primary care

Nicholas Gladstone, Chioma Onyedinma-Ndubueze and Nova Corcoran

---

NMC Standards of Proficiency for Registered Nurses

Platform 1: Being an accountable professional

Registered nurses act in the best interests of people, putting them first and providing nursing care that is person-centred, safe and compassionate. They act professionally at all times and use their knowledge and experience to make evidence-based decisions about care. They communicate effectively, are role models for others, and are accountable for their actions. Registered nurses continually reflect on their practice and keep abreast of new emerging developments in nursing, health and care.

At the point of registration, the registered nurse will be able to:

1.1 understand and act in accordance with the Code (2015): Professional standards of practice and behaviour for nurses and midwives, and fulfil all registration requirements;

1.10 demonstrate resilience and emotional intelligence and be capable of explaining the rationale that influences their judgements and decisions in routine, complex and challenging situations;

1.11 communicate effectively using a range of skills and strategies with colleagues and people at all stages of life and with a range of mental, physical, cognitive and behavioural health challenges;

1.12 demonstrate the skills and abilities required to support people at all stages of life who are emotionally or physically vulnerable;

1.13 demonstrate the skills and abilities required to develop, manage and maintain appropriate relationships with people, their families, carers and colleagues;

1.14 provide and promote non-discriminatory, person-centred and sensitive care at all times, reflecting on people's values and beliefs, diverse backgrounds, cultural characteristics, language requirements, needs and preferences, taking account of any need for adjustments.

Platform 2: Promoting health and preventing ill health

Registered nurses play a key role in improving and maintaining the mental, physical and behavioural health and well-being of people, families, communities and populations. They support and enable people at all stages of life and in all care settings to make informed choices about how to manage health challenges in order to maximise their quality of life and improve health outcomes. They are actively involved in the prevention of and protection against disease and ill health and engage in public health, community development and global health agendas, and in the reduction of health inequalities.

At the point of registration, the registered nurse will be able to:

2.7 understand and explain the contribution of social influences, health literacy, individual circumstances, behaviours and lifestyle choices to mental, physical and behavioural health outcomes;

2.10 provide information in accessible ways to help people understand and make decisions about their health, life choices, illness and care.

Platform 3: Assessing needs and planning care

Assessing needs and planning care Registered nurses prioritise the needs of people when assessing and reviewing their mental, physical, cognitive, behavioural, social and spiritual needs. They use information obtained during assessments to identify the priorities and requirements for person-centred and evidence-based nursing interventions and support. They work in partnership with people to develop person-centred care plans that take into account their circumstances, characteristics and preferences.

At the point of registration, the registered nurse will be able to:

3.4 understand and apply a person-centred approach to nursing care, demonstrating shared assessment, planning, decision making and goal setting when working with people, their families, communities and populations of all ages;

3.15 demonstrate the ability to work in partnership with people, families and carers to continuously monitor, evaluate and reassess the effectiveness of all agreed nursing care plans and care, sharing decision making and readjusting agreed goals, documenting progress and decisions made.

Chapter aims

After reading this chapter, you should be able to:

- outline the philosophy of person-centred care and highlight how this affects nursing practice and care outcomes;
- explain how key principles of the Nursing and Midwifery Council Code (2018) provide a core framework for our professional practice including assistant nurse practitioners;
- define the core values that underpin nursing and recognise their application to person-centred nursing practice;
- highlight the challenges to contemporary nursing and relate these to recognised core values.

Introduction

This chapter looks at person-centred care and asks you to think of what person-centred care means and how it is delivered in nursing. It helps you to consider how you can provide this essential element of care to the patients and their families you will encounter. It uses policy and models of care to help you to understand how you can deliver person-centred care while valuing the individual and how the care environment can influence the care we provide. The chapter ends with looking at how you can plan the care for a patient.

Read the case study below and think how your own values and those of others may impact on delivering person-centred care.

Case study: Beth

You are caring for Beth, a 35-year-old high school teacher. Beth is six weeks pregnant and was admitted due to complications regarding her pregnancy after attempting suicide. You later learn that she has been in the news for having a sexual relationship with one of her male students. Some of the staff on the ward are making judgemental remarks about her, such as they won't let her near their children and that she should not be trusted with young people, and how she abused her position as a teacher. Through caring for Beth, you learn that she had a troubled childhood and was physically and emotionally abused. The newspapers have been alerted to her admission and are ringing the ward and also roaming outside the hospital. Beth tells you that she is embarrassed by the publicity, but that she and the student are in love with each other, but no one seems to understand.

Activity 7.1   Reflection

Consider how your colleagues', society's and your own values can impact on the care of a patient.

An outline answer is provided at the end of the chapter.

Background

Caring is a central part of nursing practice, and the relationship between the patient and nurse is an important part of nursing care (Chapman, 2017). The concept of person-centredness within nursing has long been considered an important part of nursing care delivery (Bell et al., 2015), and it has the *capacity to make a critical difference to the care experience of patients and staff* (McCance et al., 2013, p1). Improving the experience that a patient has is not just about good clinical care, it is also about putting the patient at the centre of the delivery of care (McConnell et al., 2016).

The medical profession coined the term 'person-centredness' based on the philosophy of American psychologist Carl Rogers (Rogers, 1951). Rogers recognised the importance of compassion, caring, empathy, sensitivity and active listening in the promotion of optimal human growth. The term 'person-centred' is often used in a similar way to phrases such as 'client-centred', 'patient-centred' and 'patient-focused', leading to the lack of a standard definition (Ross et al., 2015). Despite any clear meaning, policies and frameworks continue to demand that healthcare professionals place the patient at the heart of all care provision and clinical decision-making. Activity 7.2 is designed to help you explore the concept of person-centredness.

Activity 7.2   Critical thinking

- What is the difference between a patient and a person?
- How do you define person-centredness?
- How does the NMC *Code* explore person-centred care?

An outline answer is provided at the end of the chapter.

In the next sections, we will look at how policy can influence person-centred care and also define the term.

Person-centred care and healthcare policy

Having considered a definition for person-centred care in Activity 7.2, we now look at how this affects healthcare policy. In 1997, the Department of Health launched reforms calling for the NHS to undergo change in a bid to offer a personalised service to patients that was 'patient-centred' (DH, 1997). The Quality Framework (DH, 1998) was developed in an attempt to ensure quality care provision in all areas of the NHS and deliver a service designed around the needs of the patient. Further initiatives included the Health and Social Care Bill (2001) that called for the greater involvement of patients and the public in all aspects of healthcare to promote change and improvement. From this philosophy, NICE (2006) embraced the principles of person-centred care instructing all acute NHS Trusts to provide services that address the personal, social, mental and physical health needs of individuals with dementia who use acute hospital facilities for any reason (NICE, 2006, p11).

NICE have produce additional guidance in different areas of nursing practice – for example, *patient experience within adult NHS services* (NICE, 2012) includes a focus on knowing the patient as an individual, tailoring healthcare services for each patient, and continuity of care and relationships. The NHS Long Term Plan was launched in 2019 and makes plans for health provisions over the next 10 years. It focuses on enabling everyone to get the best start in life, helping communities to live well and helping people to age well. All of these will incorporate some aspect of patient-centred care.

In 2010, the World Health Organization (WHO) released a framework on an integrated, people-centred health service that details its own vision for the future with the provision of care that is coordinated around patients' needs, and respects their preferences while being safe, effective, timely, affordable and of acceptable quality (WHO, 2010). Therefore, as a framework and a move towards quality care provision, person-centred care takes into consideration a service user's needs, preferences and strengths. Service users should have the opportunity to make informed choices and decisions about their treatment and care that reflect a partnership and relationship between themselves and health and social care practitioners. Partnership working is central to the delivery of person-centred care at all levels and involves balancing health promotion and patient involvement in all aspects of health and social care from primary through to tertiary.

Defining person-centred care

NHS England (2012) sets out core values in the form of the 6Cs – Care, Compassion, Competence, Communication, Courage and Commitment. These values have been embedded across healthcare, as they are directly relevant to all healthcare workers, including doctors, nurses, allied health professionals and social workers (King's Fund, 2012). It is important to empower healthcare workers across the UK to embrace the 6Cs in order to ensure that they take an approach to care that is motivated by compassion. Positive social interaction developed through effective communication is described as the cornerstone to effective person-centred care (Manley et al., 2011). Other authors argue for multiple concepts that are important for achieving person-centred care. For example, Galloway (2011) notes elements such as effective communication, involvement of the patient, being an advocate for patients, trust and honesty, and considering the patient as a whole (holism).

Nurses who strive to provide person-centred care must be self-aware. This means that you must be able to identify your own values and bring them in alignment with the NMC *Code* and the key tenets of person-centred care. These are prioritising people, practising effectively, practising safely and promoting professional image and trust (NMC, 2015).

Following consultation on the revised NMC code of conduct (NMC, 2015), the Health Foundation reaffirmed the assertion that nurses and midwives must work in partnership with patients in a person-centred manner. The Health Foundation (2014) suggests four key concepts that combine to make person-centred care a reality. These are:

- respect and holism;
- power and empowerment;
- choice and autonomy;
- empathy and compassion.

In Activity 7.3, you are asked to reflect on the four concepts of person-centred care discussed earlier. In this activity, you need to think critically about health literacy, health promotion and how you can offer person-centred care.

Activity 7.3 Reflection

Part 1

How might you make some of the four concepts a reality in your own nursing practice when you are working with others?

Part 2

Find out more about health literacy and write about how this affects care provision and health promotion and person-centred care.

You can start by accessing the Health Education England website. You can find this under Useful websites at the end of the chapter.

An outline answer is provided at the end of the chapter.

Having considered Activity 7.3 regarding health literacy and health promotion, we now turn to models of care and look at how they can be used to offer person-centred care.

Models of person-centred care

Being person-centred is not just a one-off change, but an ongoing activity (McCance and McCormack, 2017), thus a number of theories and models have been designed to help guide person-centred care delivery. Although these models differ in approach, they all share a focus on a more 'holistic' approach to care, meaning that they take into consideration a broad variety of factors that influence the whole person in the care process. Some of these factors are outside traditional biomedical models of care – for example, including emphasis on patient autonomy and capability, or making the primary focus the patient (rather than the illness) are not centred in a traditional biomedical model of care where the 'expert' knows best.

Four models or frameworks are discussed here: the Planetree Model (2012), the Gothenburg Model (2011), McCormack and McCance's Person-centred Nursing Framework (2006), and the Valuing People Framework (Alzheimer's Australia, 2014). These models have been chosen as they provide a broad overview of the principles of person-centred care, with the Planetree Model having been used for over 40 years.

The Planetree Model

The Planetree Model was developed in the USA in 1978 by Angela Thieriot. The model advocates a collaborative approach to care delivery that highlights the need for inter-professional teamwork and the development of a supportive organisational culture (i.e. the hospital environment) for patients, their families, and nursing and medical staff. The model views collaborative practice as the foundation of patient/person-centred care and promotes the need for the patient to be involved in all aspects of clinical decision-making during illness and recovery.

The Gothenburg Model of person-centred care

The Gothenburg Model proposes the need for three 'simple routines' to initiate, integrate and safeguard person-centred care in daily clinical practice (Britten et al. 2017): the patient narrative, collaborative practice and safeguarding collaborative practice. The patient narrative is the patient's personal account of their illness and the effect this has on their daily life. Collaborative practice is the shared decision-making process with patients, healthcare staff and relatives working together to achieve an agreed goal. Safeguarding collaborative practice considers the preferences and values of the patient and their family, and subsequently informs decision-making.

McCormack and McCance's Person-Centred Nursing Framework

McCormack and McCance (2006) developed a framework. Their model uses three constructs that helped form the basis of the Person-Centred Nursing Framework (2006). It is particularly useful as a tool to help healthcare practitioners identify barriers to change.

The framework identifies four key concepts (see Figure 7.1) that are important to achieving person-centred nursing:

- Care prerequisites that focus on the characteristics and qualities of the nurse.
- The care environment, which focuses on the context in which care is delivered.
- Person-centred care delivery and processes that focus on a range of activities.
- Anticipated care outcomes resulting from effective person-centred nursing.

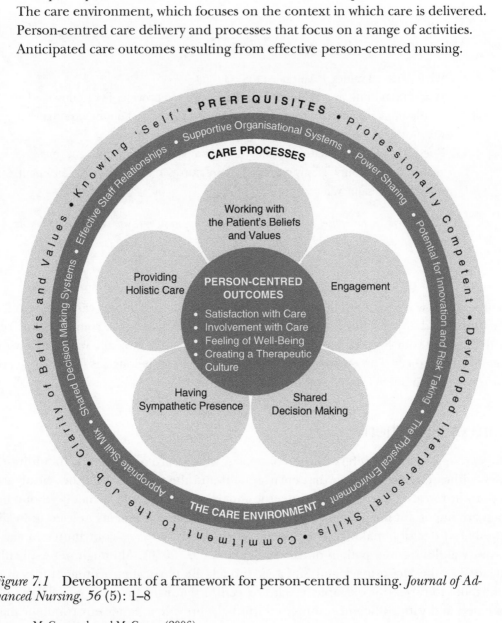

Figure 7.1 Development of a framework for person-centred nursing. *Journal of Advanced Nursing, 56* (5): 1–8

Source: McCormack and McCance (2006).

Care prerequisites

Care prerequisites focus on the attributes of a nurse – for example, the professional competence and experience of a nurse and the skills that they have, including knowledge and communication skills. They also incorporate the values and beliefs of a nurse. Other elements such as commitment to the job and the ability to know the 'self' are reflected in this section. These elements have an impact on the nurse's ability to make decisions and prioritise care in practice. In Activity 7.4, you will be asked to consider some of these prerequisites.

Activity 7.4   Reflection

- What personal values do you need to be a nurse?
- How do you think your values influence the care you provide? For example, what do you think is important to you and how might this impact on the care that you will provide?
- Does a nurse have to share the same values as a patient? Depending on your answer, can you think of any examples where nurses and patients share or might not share the same values?

As this is a reflexive exercise, no outline answer is provided, but you can revisit Chapter 1 for some ideas.

Getting to know your patient in terms of their life outside their illness can help to offer person-centred approaches to care. For example, if you learn that your patient likes gardening and your hospital has a gardening project, you can look at a way of involving them in this project. The environment to which the person belongs as well as the care environment can impact on person-centred care.

Care environment

The care environment refers to the context in which care is delivered. In addition, the healthcare workers within that environment and the skill mix that they bring are important to care delivery. Shared decision-making and an appropriately resourced team are important for patient-centred care. In addition, the systems needed to facilitate shared decision-making. A conducive environment of care contributes to early recovery and improved patient outcomes (Eaton et al., 2016). Although not explicitly included in the McCormack and McCance model, the physical environment may also contribute to care – for example, a ward or centre that is fit for purpose, that is well designed and with sufficient resources – will help provide a better environment that allows people to work more efficiently.

Care processes

By adopting the nursing processes and a problem-solving approach to care, a nurse should be able to work with the patient and their family to negotiate a plan of care. This plan should take into consideration the patient's beliefs, values, needs, relations, preferences, cognitive ability and willingness to negotiate a care plan that is based on shared decision-making (McCormack and McCance, 2010). This is reflected in the government white paper *Equity and Excellence: Liberating the NHS* (2012) that details the government's vision of patients being placed at the heart of the NHS and a need for shared decision-making, with the philosophy 'No decision about me without me'.

Case study: Abdul

Abdul is a 29-year-old patient in your care. He is visited by his boyfriend, Calvin (they share a flat together), but his family is unaware of his same-sex relationship and thinks Calvin is his friend. It is difficult for Abdul as he wants to include Calvin in his care decisions, but his family can be overbearing at times and ignores Calvin. You overheard a colleague saying that Abdul is living a double life and this will end badly.

Activity 7.5   Reflection

After reading the sections below, consider how you can provide person-centred care to Abdul. Think about how you can make a connection with the patient.

An outline answer is provided at the end of the chapter.

To be able to understand the patient as a person, a comprehensive assessment should be carried out to ensure a broad understanding of their needs and the challenges they may face. This includes not only the current illness and the medical needs of the patient, but the environment outside the hospital and the community in which that patient lives. There are assessment frameworks such as Roper (1976) or Orem (1980) that can provide a structure for your information gathering, which may help your communication skills. This is an essential prerequisite for person-centred care provision and the development of a connection with the patient as a person. Further assessment of the identified problems may also be required and can be facilitated through the use of a specific risk-assessment tool relevant to the problem (Barrett et al., 2012).

Care outcomes

Based on person-centred goals and effective nursing care, care outcomes should be measured from a person's or family's perspective. As with the term 'person-centred', there is no standard definition for a 'care outcome', making it difficult to distinguish what exactly should be measured or how.

Evidence suggests that when a person-centred approach is applied within the nursing process, as detailed within the NMC *Code* (2015), it makes its adoption in nursing practice more achievable. This assertion is confirmed in a study by Clissett et al. (2013) who found that better or improved patient and carer outcomes were associated with a person-centred care approach.

Case study: Olatunde

Olatunde is of African heritage and has been admitted to your ward for surgery. On assessment, his family tells you that he has started getting forgetful lately. When you ask them to describe his forgetfulness, they give examples of not remembering where he placed his house keys and sometimes they find items of his clothes in the refrigerator. His family tells you that he is a leader in their local community and provides advice and support to other members of the African community. Your mentor suggests that he may have early onset dementia and would like to refer him to the dementia team for an assessment. His family tells you that dementia does not exist and that they believe it is evil spirits sent upon him as a result of other people's envy of his upstanding position in their community.

Activity 7.6   Critical thinking

After reading the next section, think of how you can value an individual and their cultural beliefs.

An outline answer is provided at the end of this chapter.

The Valuing People Framework

Another philosophy that encompasses the essence of person-centred care is the Valuing People Framework, which was developed by Alzheimer's Australia (2014) and the Australian Department of Social Services. This recognises the importance of person-centredness in the delivery of care for individuals diagnosed with dementia living in the community. In an attempt to promote person-centred care, the framework promotes valuing and appreciating the individual as a human being with moral worth as a key principle. Person-centred care is enhanced when a therapeutic relationship is established with the service user, in which they are able to engage in all or some aspects of their care. This approach takes into consideration the person's beliefs (or lack of), values and strengths. Through empowerment and provision of information, the service user is allowed to make autonomous decisions and informed choices to achieve agreed goals (DH, 2005).

Brooke et al. (2017) suggest that our culture has an impact on the way we understand dementia, and the care and support that we give to those with dementia. They suggest that migrant workers from outside a host country might need support with communication skills to help provide culturally competent healthcare for those with dementia. In Activity 7.7 you are asked to explore your views on dementia through reflection.

Activity 7.7   Critical thinking

- Why do you think people might have different views of dementia?
- How do you think your view of dementia might affect the care that you provide?

An outline answer is provided at the end of this chapter.

Challenges in current practice

Despite a number of policies and frameworks, there is still substantial evidence that demonstrates substandard care provision and poor patient engagement within patient-centred practice. Inquiries and subsequent reports by Keogh (2013), Francis (2013) and Andrews (2014) all highlight significant failings in care delivery and the consequent suffering of patients. The notion of person-centredness can be undermined by a number of challenges – for example, how a workplace culture can allow and may reinforce poor standards of care and the subsequent disengagement by staff within these workplaces, or not maintaining staffing levels to provide optimum care. Other challenges include training around diversity and inclusive practice, clinical updates to ensure that staff are supported to offer the care required or working equipment. Some of these reports – for example, Francis (2013) – and the media coverage of failings detailed within them, demonstrate that there has been a significant change in both nursing regulation and care delivery in recent years. However, barriers and challenges to patient-centred practice still remain.

Barriers to implementing person-centred care are numerous. They include the healthcare environment, the processes, resources and systems within healthcare, the health professional and the patient. These vary across different settings and within different healthcare systems. For example, in primary healthcare, barriers may include workload, time and resources (Rubio-Valera et al., 2014). In an intensive care unit, the emotional and physical demands of critical care can act as a barrier and compromise the ability of nurses to provide patient care (Jakimowicz et al., 2017). In an emergency department, nurses may have little control over the environment with the pressures of getting patients through the department (McConnell et al., 2016). In addition, the attitudes, values, personal qualities and knowledge of both the healthcare worker and the patient will influence the care process. This makes addressing the barriers to providing patient-centred care challenging, as no one solution will fit everyone.

Organisational culture

As detailed in the Francis Report (2013), person-centred care should be promoted and informed by the leadership of every healthcare system. When change emanates from the top – i.e. managers or chief executives – staff can then promote change at ground level in the wards, clinics and community settings in which they work. The organisational culture should therefore be one that humanises the experience of the patient.

Leadership style and support can have a significant impact on the promotion and delivery of person-centred care in practice. Many acute hospital settings struggle to provide care that recognises the importance of placing the person at the centre of their care and instead focus on fiscal measures such as making cost savings or financial targets. There is a need for effective leadership that will facilitate the process of person-centred nursing with support available for staff to increase their knowledge and awareness of person-centred care principles and the place of this in quality care delivery. Regular professional updates on the practice of person-centred care will only enhance staff competence in practice. The organisational culture must be such that it enables staff to achieve excellence in their practice and subsequent patient outcomes irrespective of any financial or resource constraints.

Care environment

As with organisational culture, the care environment has a significant influence on the successful implementation of person-centred care. McCance et al. (2013) argues that these two areas alongside the learning environment provide the greatest challenges to person-centred care. Hospital wards are often seen as a threat to the personal identity of a patient who may suddenly find themselves in a busy and unfamiliar environment. This threat is particularly evident in patients with learning disabilities or dementia who become unsettled and disorientated through a change in surroundings and routine (Clissett et al., 2013). For person-centred care to be successful, the care environment must be one that fosters preferred patient outcomes at all times. Time constraints and high-pressured working environments are often seen as some of the barriers to adopting and delivering person-centred care, especially in acute care settings. However, the values and behaviours involved in a person-centred care framework should reduce the impact of these constraints.

Self-awareness

Our own values and beliefs have a significant impact on the care we provide and its success or failure. Nurses must be compassionate at a time when those they care for are at their most vulnerable. Knowing the 'person' behind the 'patient' is the whole essence of person-centred care provision. This involves understanding the human 'being' in their situation. The understanding of what makes a human 'being' can be divided into four sections: being with self, being in relation, being in a social world and being in place.

Being with self

Every person has a fundamental human need to be recognised as a person with beliefs and values, seeking clarity and acceptance at the point of their need. This is central to person-centred practice (McCormack and McCance, 2010). This means taking into consideration what is important to a person – for example, what a patient thinks may have caused an illness can impact on how they then respond to medical treatment, compliance and aftercare. Cultural or religious beliefs may impact on specific care practices such as bathing, dress or food within the hospital environment.

Hafskjold et al. (2015) suggest that person-centred care should explore a patient's situation by listening and asking questions. These questions should include the discussion of care and treatment alternatives, and the provision of information by the healthcare worker. In Activity 7.8 you will be asked to think about the nursing environments that you have been in so far and delivering person-centred care.

Activity 7.8   Reflection

Think about the nursing environments you have been in so far.

- What barriers can you see to delivering the person-centred care suggested by Hafskjold et al. (2015)?
- Can you make a list of possible solutions to these barriers?

An outline answer is provided at the end of this chapter.

Activity 7.8 should help you to understand the next section, which discusses how caring for a patient involves the space and time they occupy.

Being in relation

This core concept indicates a relational connectedness with the person in receipt of nursing care. Several nurse theorists have discussed interpersonal processes that enable the development of therapeutic relationships (Peplau, 1992; Watson, 1999). All of these require knowing and valuing oneself and others, moral integrity, reflective ability, authentic engagement and sympathetic presence, as well as working in partnership with the person who is the patient. This can include building a rapport with them, through listening and asking appropriate questions to help develop the nurse–patient relationship.

Being in a social world

Every person has a 'story' that needs to be heard and understood. These narratives and biographies provide us with a picture of the person's being in the world and their interpretation of that being. Persons are constantly creating and re-creating meaning with their social world, where they have been. Respect for the person's narratives enhances quality of care provision. For example, patients may give non-medical explanations for their illness, or make sense of a long-term condition through different ways of coping. Respect for these 'stories' are important, even if you feel they conflict with modern Western medicine.

Being in place

This can be described as a mix of care environments and the recognition of the impact of these on care experiences and healing qualities. It also includes the design of buildings and space, and the potential of these to impact on care. In some environments, closer attention to building design and hospital environments can improve the care experience for patients and healthcare staff. Examples include dementia-friendly hospital settings, which have been shown to have a dramatic impact on hospital stays for those with dementia (Waller and Masterson, 2015), and new buildings that are specifically designed to maximise healthcare experiences – for example, the 'Maggie's' centres that support people with cancer are designed to be friendly and inspiring places (Maggie's, 2018).

The Johari Window

In the 1960s, American psychologists Joseph Luft and Harry Ingham developed the Johari Window (1961) to explore communication, and the views, values, beliefs and knowledge that underpin how we interact with others. The model comprises a window divided into four quadrants (see Figure 7.2 below) that signify what is known or unknown to the individual, and known or unknown to others (Luft, 1961).

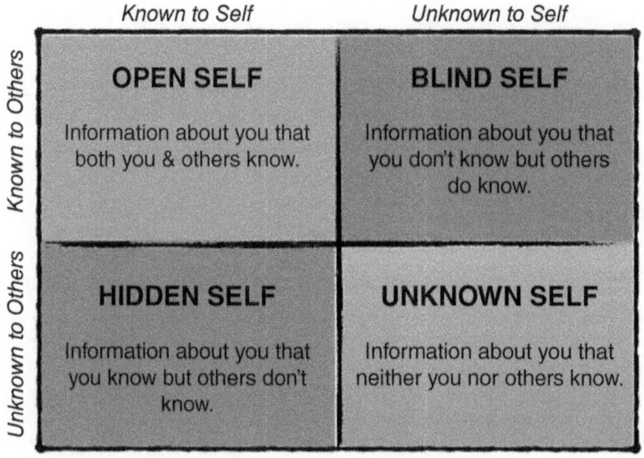

	Known to Self	*Unknown to Self*
Known to Others	**OPEN SELF** Information about you that both you & others know.	**BLIND SELF** Information about you that you don't know but others do know.
Unknown to Others	**HIDDEN SELF** Information about you that you know but others don't know.	**UNKNOWN SELF** Information about you that neither you nor others know.

Figure 7.2   The Johari Window (adapted from Luft, 1961, p6)

Luft and Ingham claim that by gaining an understanding into how others see us – both good and bad – we can become more self-aware and consider how our behaviour and values influence how we communicate. This concurs with the NMC Standards (2015) that state:

All nurses must build partnerships and therapeutic relationships through safe, effective and non-discriminatory communication. They must take account of individual differences, capabilities and needs.

(p15)

It also states:

All nurses must use a range of communication skills and technologies to support person-centred care and enhance quality and safety. They must ensure people receive all the information they need in a language and manner that allows them to make informed choices and share decision making. They must recognise when language interpretation or other communication support is needed and know how to obtain it.

(p15)

By gaining an understanding of how we act, think and behave, we can increase how open we are to ourselves, our colleagues and, most importantly, our patients.

The nursing process

To be able to provide care that captures the true essence of person-centredness, the nurse must be able to identify what the individual's needs are and develop a strategy on how these can be met. This method is referred to as the 'nursing process' and uses a structured approach to identify actual and potential problems, and plan the delivery of person-specific care. Based on the philosophies of Orlando (1961) and Petro-Yura and Walsh (1967), the nursing process consists of a five-step cyclical model. These are outlined in Figure 7.3 and are explained in more detail below.

Although each of the steps of the nursing process are viewed separately, they are not independent of one another and have overlapping connections and steps that inform practice and centre on the patient's needs (Carpenito-Moyet, 2007). Assessment must be comprehensive, complete, accurate and reliable to allow for a diagnosis. Diagnostic statements then inform nursing interventions, goals and outcomes, allowing for an individual, person-centred plan of care that addresses the problems that have been raised. The nursing process must be undertaken methodically and chronologically, leading from assessment through to evaluation, with no section skipped or overlooked (Carpenito-Moyet, 2007).

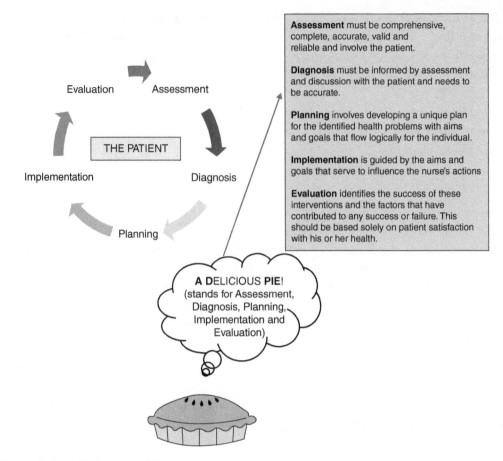

Figure 7.3 A Delicious PIE

Assessment

Assessment enables the nurse to gather information through interviewing, observing and measuring. This allows the nurse to develop a relationship with the patient that leads to the discovery of the patient's needs, wants, values and beliefs, and the many extrinsic and intrinsic factors that affect their health and well-being. Information is collected, interpreted and evaluated before any diagnoses are made and care planned. Assessment requires critical thinking skills to compare different factors and the value the patient places on these (Howartson-Jones et al., 2015).

According to Jarvis (2016), physical assessment is a vital skill used to attain information and knowledge about a patient that allows a nurse to identify and recognise any abnormalities. Through open dialogue and questioning, the nurse can gain important information, not only about the physical illness and symptoms that a patient may be presenting with, but also the sociocultural, environmental and psychological factors that contribute to the patient's 'sense of wellness'.

Chabeli (2007) asserts that while nurses focus on illness and the physiological causes of this, it is equally important to consider areas such as non-verbal communication, behaviour and mannerisms, all of which provide the nurse with cues and clues as to the patient's emotional well-being. For example, by looking at a patient, you might be able to see if they are anxious or upset. Coombs et al. (2011) agree with this assertion, stating that nursing assessment should also consider a person's social circumstances, behaviour and mental health when undertaking an assessment.

Diagnosis

Nursing diagnosis forms an integral part of the nursing process, allowing the nurse to identify the physical and psychosocial problems from the collected data, and form diagnostic statements that detail the patient's wants and needs. Creating a diagnosis requires critical thinking skills, good communication and an understanding of the patient and their situation alongside an insight into how they themselves view their health and well-being (Ackley and Ladwig, 2014). The nursing diagnosis can be undertaken with the help of classifications that act as an aide-memoire to inform clinical decision-making; examples include the North American Nursing Diagnosis Association (NANDA) nursing classification (NANDA, 2012).

Planning

Wilson et al. (2018) assert that care planning is a strategic approach to organising and preparing care based on nursing assessment and diagnosis, followed by implementation and evaluation. Within the context of person-centred care, this part of the nursing process is arguably the most important and should focus on what the patient wants and the needs they have. The patient should be central to all decision-making, with realistic goals and aims that are congruent with their expectations and perceived outcomes (Leach, 2008).

Implementation

Nursing interventions can be defined as activities and actions designed to address and meet the individual needs of the patient (Saba and Taylor, 2007). When considering each intervention, the nurse is required to work with the patient to identify what help they need to reach any goals that have been set. Additionally, the nurse is also required to ensure that any intervention is evidence-based and part of best practice rather than just traditional or routine. As previously discussed, interventions that are focused on a patient's needs and collaborative practice have been found to be more successful. The need for patient involvement reaffirms the importance of person-centred care and shared decision-making throughout the nursing process (Chabeli, 2007).

Evaluation

Evaluation in the nursing process can be described as ongoing. During the assessment, a nurse evaluates whether or not enough information has been collected to form a nursing diagnosis. The nursing diagnoses are evaluated for their correctness, and then goals and interventions are evaluated for their chance to be realistic and reachable. If they are not, plans should be developed or changed. While undertaking interventions, evaluation is needed to consider if those interventions lead to the achievement of set goals. Evaluation is important since, in the absence of evaluation, it is almost impossible to know whether the care actually helps to meet the needs of the patient. Even if an intervention is not working very well, the knowledge from evaluating the intervention can help a nurse to develop care in the future. In the case study below, you are asked to consider how you can evaluate the care provided to a patient.

Case study: Ms Turner

Ms Turner, a patient in your care, has a diagnosis of cancer of the breast, which has spread to other parts of her body. She is a registered nurse and all the staff know her as she works in the same hospital. Your mentor has asked you to plan Ms Turner's care for the day. You have done your assessment on maintaining personal hygiene and have devised the care plan.

Activity 7.9   Critical thinking

- Make a list of how you assessed the care needed for personal hygiene.
- Think about how you will evaluate the care provided.

An outline answer is provided at the end of the chapter.

Evaluation of a patient's care comes at the end of assessing, planning and implementing care, which is known as the care plan. The section below explains the components of a care plan.

Writing a plan of care

A plan of care is a document that details in a clear and concise way the care and support provided to a patient. It should be written with and agreed by the patient through the process of care planning and review (Barrett et al., 2012). Respecting patients as people and being able to include them within a care partnership is an important part of a person-centred approach.

Care planning involves:

- *Gathering and sharing information* – for example, the needs, views and wants of all concerned, including the patient and their family alongside members of the multidisciplinary team (MDT).
- A *clear and structured overview* of the patient's needs and the impact these have on their health and well-being.
- *Exploration and discussion of information and nursing diagnoses*: to provide a clear understanding of health needs, and categorise and prioritise these accordingly.
- *Goal setting*: clear aims and objectives that detail what the patient wants to achieve and how the nurse and members of the MDT can help the patient.
- *Action planning*: what is the plan, who will be responsible for it and when will it be reviewed?

Standards

Standards for care planning come from a number of sources. These include the Care Quality Commission *Essential Standards of Quality and Safety*. This requires that the assessment, planning and delivery of care is centred on a patient as an individual and considers all aspects of their individual circumstances, and their immediate and long-term needs. It also states that this should be developed with patients or those acting on their behalf, should reflect their needs, preferences and diversity, and identify risks, and how these will be managed and reviewed. In addition, plans of care, treatment and support should be implemented, flexible, regularly reviewed for their effectiveness and changed if they are found to be ineffective. They need to be kept up to date in recognition of the changing needs of the person using the service.

Where and how the care plan should be written

Where and how a care plan is written may have a major impact on how effective the care plan is. A care plan should ensure that a patient gets the same care, regardless of who is nursing that patient. It should support a patient to manage their condition, and should be developed 'with' a patient, not 'for' a patient. A care plan that is written by one person alone in an office without patient involvement may include all the key elements, but is not likely to be as effective in practice as one that is written in partnership with the person and those who are contributing to the plan. Often, concerns are expressed about the time needed to write comprehensive plans and, as a result, care plans can become jargonised shorthand for what services will do. This type of plan is unhelpful to service users, carers and staff. A sense of ownership by all those concerned – and in particular the person themselves – is vital in making the plan translate into reality, which can be promoted by:

- *Using people's own words and phrases* (familiar and comfortable language, which avoids jargon and abbreviations).
- Recognising that *care plans exist for the benefit of the service user,* and should be based around the needs of that person, not around the services available.
- *Involving the person in agreeing and writing* the care plan as much as possible, including the opportunity to sign the care plan.
- Producing the plan in a *format and style that the person is comfortable with.*
- *Being flexible* in the approach to the service user's involvement.

Content of care plans

Care plans for all service users should include:

- *Why* are we doing this? (aims)
- *What* are we planning to achieve? (outcomes)
- *How* are we going to do it? (actions)
- *Who* will do it? (responsibilities)
- *Where* will it be done? (times, locations)
- *When* will it be done by? (timescales)
- Any needs relating to *REGARDS* (Race and culture, Economic disadvantage, Gender, Age, Religion/Spirituality, disability or sexuality).

Read the case study below and consider Andrew's problems. Then write a care plan for the patient, as outlined in Activity 7.10.

Case study: Andrew

Andrew is 19 years old and has suffered fractures to his pelvis. He also has severe muscle and tissue loss to his left leg, together with a complex fracture of his tibia and fibula following a motorcycle accident. Andrew has been reviewed by the trauma and orthopaedic team who are preparing to take him for emergency surgery. The surgeons have told Andrew that they are unable to save his left leg and that he will need an above-knee amputation.

Andrew's vital signs are: temperature: 34.9°C; pulse: 109 beats per minute; respiration: 20 breaths per minute; oxygen saturation: 95% on 15l O_2 via a Hudson non-rebreathing oxygen mask; blood pressure: 89/68 mmHg; AVPU: alert and in pain.

Past medical history: none.

Activity 7.10   Critical thinking

Initial assessment of Andrew has shown that he has multiple fractures and is in severe pain. Using the ADPIE tool, write a care plan showing how you would assess and treat Andrew's pain and evaluate the care you have provided. Remember that your goals need to be achievable, with clear aims and objectives.

Assessment	Diagnosis	Plan (goal)	Intervention	Evaluation

An outline answer is provided at the end of the chapter.

We hope that from reading this chapter and working through the activities, you have developed a better sense of person-centred care and that this will help you to develop your practice as a nurse.

Chapter summary

Person-centred care is an important skill within nursing practice, and one that can improve patient outcomes. This chapter has described the concept of person-centred care and identified why person-centred care is important to nursing practice. It has given suggestions of ways for you to reflect on your own values and beliefs, and how these might impact on the care that you provide as a nurse. The chapter has also outlined the challenges to achieving person-centred care and discussed the different ways that nursing care can work to be more person-centred. It has identified core principles within key policies and the NMC *Code* (2015) that are important to person-centred care. Finally, this chapter has outlined the nursing process and given suggestions for writing a care plan that is grounded in person-centred care.

Activities: Brief outline answers

Activity 7.1   Reflection (p145)

See Figure 7.4. The answers given in the framework are not exhaustive but are only indicative.

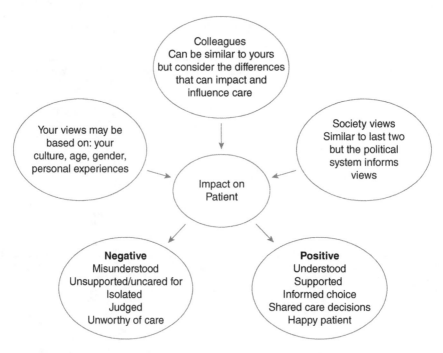

Figure 7.4   Possible impacts of values on a patient

Activity 7.2   Critical thinking (p145)

The word 'patient' comes from the Latin *patiens*, from *patior*, meaning to suffer or bear. However, in healthcare a patient is someone who is receiving care or treatment for some form of illness. A person is an individual who has the ability to make decisions concerning morality, reasons, judgements and who has a consciousness. A person usually belongs to a cultural group whose practices and beliefs influence their being.

Person-centredness can be defined as focusing on the care the individual needs rather than on the service. For example, in our opening case study, Beth may need to have medical examinations (a service), as well as person-centred care through listening to her and offering care that is appropriate to her situation. In person-centredness, you will need to acknowledge the individual's desires, values, family situations, social circumstances and lifestyles, seeing the person as an individual, and working together to develop appropriate solutions.

The NMC is putting patients and their families at the core of their work. For example, the NMC is adopting a new person-centred approach to fitness to practise. It ensures that patients and families are treated with compassion and respect, and that their concerns about nurses and midwives are properly addressed and listened to. The NMC is also improving the way it communicates with people to make sure that it is clear, empathetic, helpful and easy to understand. *Future Nurse: Standards of Proficiency for Registered Nurses* (NMC, 2018) emphasises person-centred care as part of evidence-based care that is compassionate.

Activity 7.3   Reflection (p147)

Part 1

- *Respect and holism*: show respect for Beth as a person, which includes placing your own values aside and viewing her in a non-judgemental way. This means ignoring the newspaper reports and comments from your colleagues. Holistic care will involve addressing Beth's mental health as well as her physical health; therefore, you may want to make a referral to the hospital mental health or psychological services team.
- *Power and empowerment*: as a student nurse, Beth is in your care and there will be a power relationship as she is your patient and you will be making decisions regarding her care. You will need to reflect on how you can make value-free judgements that offer the best possible care to her. You may also want to look at how to get Beth to take ownership for some of her care through empowering her. You may do this by providing her with information on services available or directing her to online literature that can help her make informed decisions.
- *Choice and autonomy*: during your nurse education, you will hear the terms 'informed choice', 'informed decision' or 'informed consent'. These phrases indicate that the individual or patient was provided with information and, based on this, can make a choice or decision on the care they need. For example, in the case study with Beth, you can provide her with options on mental health support and she can make an informed choice on how she would like her care to be delivered. Similarly, autonomy goes together with choice, as Beth will have control over how her care is planned and can influence the pathway for her care.
- *Empathy and compassion*: empathy is not to be confused with sympathy. Empathy is concerned with being able to understand and share how your patient may be feeling about their situation. In the case of Beth, you can show empathy by listening to her, understanding how her past may impact on her present situation and being sensitive to her needs. You can show compassion by understanding the place that Beth is in psychologically. Using therapeutic touch can help to convey compassion. Also, use of non-verbal communication such as nodding to show understanding or using facial gestures as appropriate can convey compassion. Taking time to sit with Beth and discuss her care and options of other services available to her is also a way of providing compassionate care.

Part 2

- Look around your care environment and identify opportunities for using health literacy.
- Try to identify the barriers to health literacy.
- Make a list of how you can overcome the barriers you identified.

Activity 7.5   Reflection (p151)

- You can discuss with Abdul how he would like his care to be offered. This is part of the care planning process and you will learn how to do this from your mentors.
- You and your mentor can ask Abdul how much he would like Calvin to be involved in his care. You can discuss areas such as how much information to share with Calvin and whether he wants Calvin to be his next-of-kin contact.
- Areas of care that Calvin can be involved in are feeding, dressing and helping Abdul to maintain personal care such as washing and shaving.
- After focusing on his partner, you can ask questions about his family's involvement in his care in a similar way.
- Together with your mentor, identify what Abdul likes to eat so you can offer him food to his taste. You can also find out what he likes doing as a hobby and find ways to make this part of his care – for example, he may like playing football and although he cannot play, you can arrange for him to watch a game on television with other patients.
- You need to remember to approach Abdul's living circumstances with sensitivity, especially as his family is unaware of his same-sex relationship; you must also maintain patient confidentiality.

Activity 7.6   Critical thinking (p152)

Moorley et al. (2016) advise that you should always acknowledge your patient's culture when caring for them. It is important that you consider and understand your patient's and their family's beliefs and practices. Although this may contradict medical and nursing knowledge, you need to listen to your patient and find a medium between acknowledging their culture and care that is beneficial to them. There may be other professionals you can use to help you explain and adapt care to meet the patient's needs. Remember, some cultures may require gender-matched care – for example, only females to care for female patients and vice versa. Other areas include food – some cultural groups hold specific beliefs about food types and the impact on their health. You should also consider prayer times or religious practices and how you can incorporate these into the patient's care.

Activity 7.7   Critical thinking (p153)

The reasons listed below of people's different views of dementia are not exhaustive.

- Different views can be based on poor or low level of health literacy.
- There may be cultural beliefs and practices that influence the view of dementia.
- The patient may have a language barrier or cognitive disability.
- The person may have a low level of knowledge or may not have encountered dementia before.
- Some people may have experience of engaging with people with dementia and this may influence their views.

Reflecting on your own view of dementia and how it may affect the care that you provide, you could consider your personal and professional values, and experience of working with people with dementia. You could also consider how your own culture influences your views.

Activity 7.8   Reflection (p155)

This answer is based on your experience, but some barriers may be lack of resources, the physical layout of the ward, lack of staff to help provide the care needed; time may also be a barrier.

Again, this is based on your experience. Some tips are that you may want to involve other members of the team to help – for example, an occupational therapist may be able to assist. You may want to look at organising breaktimes so that you maximise the time you have and colleagues around you to support. You may be able to reorganise the patient's bed area to maximise space.

Activity 7.9   Critical thinking (p160)

It is always good to start by asking the patient how independent they are in caring for their need.

Ask if they can clean their own teeth, brush their hair and how much can they do to wash themselves. These questions will give you the answer to how much assistance you will need to give.

You can then ask whether the patient uses soap on their face, or have they got their own skin care products. Other areas include water temperature, ability to dress independently or needing help.

Based on your assessment and overall patient risk assessment, you will need to decide if you can deliver the care on your own or whether you will need another healthcare professional to help you.

To evaluate the care provided:

- When possible, you should always ask the patient or their family if they are happy with the episode of care.
- Assess if you provided the care you set out to give – for example, did the patient's teeth get cleaned, was their skin moisturised?
- By using this approach, you can also find out if the way you delivered the care was the best to meet the patient's need and this will help you to modify or improve the care.

Activity 7.10   Critical thinking (p163)

The following example focuses on pain.

Assessment	Diagnosis	Plan (goal)	Intervention	Evaluation
Pain	Multiple fractures	That the patient will be pain free.	Assess the level, location and type of pain using a pain-scoring tool.	Evaluate the effect of the medication by assessing the patient's pain using the pain tool.
			Ask the patient what usually relieves their pain. Apart from medication, they may have other techniques they use – for example, mindfulness.	Ask the patient if the level of pain is still the same or whether it is better or worse.
			Look up the WHO pain ladder.	Evaluate by asking the patient if repositioning helped.
			With your mentor, discuss with the medical team the pain relief needed and ensure that it is administered by an appropriate healthcare professional.	
			You can reposition the patient to help ease the pain.	

Further reading

Brooker, D and Latham, I (2015) *Person-centred Dementia Care: Making Services Better with the VIPS Framework.* London: Jessica Kingsley.

This book will give you a deeper understanding of how to provide person-centred dementia care. It explores issues related to person-centred dementia care and how services can enable individuals with dementia to live well.

NHS England (2016) *Personalised Care and Support Planning Handbook: The Journey to Person-centred Care: Core Information.* Leeds: Care and Support Planning Working Group and Coalition for Collaborative Care.

This handbook provides information on how to deliver personalised care and support person-centred care planning.

Price, B (2019) *Delivering Person-centred Care in Nursing.* London: SAGE.

This book looks at delivering effective and responsive care that is person centred. It uses a range of case studies in a variety of nursing settings. It provides guidance for transforming your ideas of person-centred care into a reality.

Tee, S (ed.) (2016) *Person-centred Approaches in Healthcare: A Handbook for Nurses and Midwives.* Milton Keynes: Open University Press.

This book provides a comprehensive overview of different approaches to person-centred care in diverse settings.

Useful websites

Use this link for Activity 7.2:

https://hee.nhs.uk/our-work/hospitals-primary-community-care/population-health-prevention/health-literacy

The Health Foundation person-centred care resource:

https://personcentredcare.health.org.uk/overview-of-person-centred-care/what-person-centred-care

Health Education England Person-centred care:

www.hee.nhs.uk/our-work/person-centred-care

Future Nurse: Standards of Proficiency for Registered Nurses

www.nmc.org.uk/globalassets/sitedocuments/education-standards/print-friendly-future-nurse-proficiencies.pdf

Social Care Institute for Excellence Person-centred Care

www.scie.org.uk/person-centred-care:

Chapter 8

Understanding pharmacology and introducing medicines management

Debra Jones and Rosetta West

NMC Standards of Proficiency for Registered Nurses

Platform 1: Being an accountable professional

Registered nurses act in the best interests of people, putting them first and providing nursing care that is person-centred, safe and compassionate. They act professionally at all times and use their knowledge and experience to make evidence-based decisions about care. They communicate effectively, are role models for others, and are accountable for their actions. Registered nurses continually reflect on their practice and keep abreast of new and emerging developments in nursing, health and care.

At the point of registration, the registered nurse will be able to:

1.1 understand and act in accordance with the *Code* (2015): Professional standards of practice and behaviour for nurses and midwives, and fulfil all registration requirements;

1.3 understand and apply the principles of courage, transparency and the professional duty of candour, recognising and reporting any situations, behaviours or errors that could result in poor care outcomes;

1.8 demonstrate the knowledge, skills and ability to think critically when applying evidence and drawing on experience to make evidence informed decisions in all situations;

1.15 demonstrate the numeracy, literacy, digital and technological skills required to meet the needs of people in their care to ensure safe and effective nursing practice.

Platform 3: Assessing needs and planning care

Registered nurses prioritise the needs of people when assessing and reviewing their mental, physical, cognitive, behavioural, social and spiritual needs. They use information obtained during assessments to identify the priorities and requirements for person-centred and evidence-based nursing interventions and support. They work in partnership with people to develop person-centred care plans that take into account their circumstances, characteristics and preferences.

At the point of registration, the registered nurse will be able to:

3.2   demonstrate and apply knowledge of body systems and homeostasis, human anatomy and physiology, biology, genomics, pharmacology and social and behavioural sciences when undertaking full and accurate person-centred nursing assessments and developing appropriate care plans;

3.4   understand and apply a person-centred approach to nursing care, demonstrating shared assessment, planning, decision making and goal setting when working with people, their families, communities and populations of all ages;

3.5   demonstrate the ability to accurately process all information gathered during the assessment process to identify needs for individualised nursing care and develop person-centred evidence-based plans for nursing interventions with agreed goals;

3.6   effectively assess a person's capacity to make decisions about their own care and to give or withhold consent;

3.8   understand and apply the relevant laws about mental capacity for the country in which you are practising when making decisions in relation to people who do not have capacity.

Platform 4: Providing and evaluating care

Registered nurses take the lead in providing evidence-based, compassionate and safe nursing interventions. They ensure that the care they provide and delegate is person-centred and of a consistently high standard. They support people of all ages in a range of care settings. They work in partnership with people, families and carers to evaluate whether care is effective and the goals of care have been met in line with their wishes, preferences and desired outcomes.

At the point of registration, the registered nurse will be able to:

4.3   demonstrate the knowledge, communication and relationship management skills required to provide people, families and carers with accurate information that meets their needs before, during and after a range of interventions.

Platform 6: Improving safety and quality of care

Registered nurses make a key contribution to the continuous monitoring and quality improvement of care and treatment in order to enhance health outcomes and people's experience of nursing and related care. They assess risks to safety or experience and take appropriate action to manage those, putting the best interests, needs and preferences of people first.

At the point of registration, the registered nurse will be able to:

6.1 understand and apply the principles of health and safety legislation and regulations and maintain safe work and care environments;

6.3 comply with local and national frameworks, legislation and regulations for assessing, managing and reporting risks, ensuring the appropriate action is taken;

6.8 demonstrate an understanding of how to identify, report and critically reflect on near misses, critical incidents, major incidents and serious adverse events in order to learn from them and influence their future practice.

Annexe B: Nursing procedures

At the point of registration, the registered nurse will be able to safely demonstrate the following procedures:

11. procedural competencies required for best practice, evidence-based medicines administration and optimisation;

11.1 carry out initial and continued assessments of people receiving care and their ability to self-administer their own medications;

11.4 undertake accurate drug calculations for a range of medications;

11.6 exercise professional accountability in ensuring the safe administration of medicines to those receiving care.

Chapter aims

After reading this chapter, you will be able to:

- understand what the body does to a drug: explain the term pharmacokinetics and recognise some of the basic principles involved;
- understand what a drug does to the body: explain the term pharmacodynamics and recognise some of the basic principles involved;
- relate the principles of pharmacodynamics and pharmacokinetics to medication commonly encountered in clinical practice;
- identify and understand the most common routes of drug administration;
- describe some of the processes involved in safe and effective drug administration;
- outline some of the factors that contribute to medication errors in clinical practice;
- be competent in basic medicines calculations relating to tablets, capsules and injections, including converting units.

Introduction

Case study: Chinyere

Chinyere is a first-year adult nursing student working on her second clinical placement on a busy medical ward. She is working alongside her mentor, Matt, caring for six patients. During the drug round a patient asks Matt about one of his medications which he believes is new. Matt politely informs the patient that he will check the patient's medical and nursing notes, and come back when he has finished the drug round to speak to him and answer his questions.

After consulting the medical and nursing notes, Matt notices that the patient has recently been diagnosed with gastro oesophageal reflux disease (GORD) and started on a course of omeprazole. Matt locates a copy of the *British National Formulary* (BNF) as a resource, and both Matt and Chinyere sit down with the patient to listen to his questions and concerns.

Matt explains to the patient how omeprazole works to reduce the symptoms of GORD and informs the patient when he should take the medication. He highlights the importance of taking the drug daily for the duration of the course and not to break open the capsule as this can reduce its effectiveness. Matt also explains some of the most common side effects associated with omeprazole and why he should report these to the nursing staff. Finally, Chinyere suggests finding a patient information leaflet regarding omeprazole for him to read.

Later in the day Matt and Chinyere reflect on this episode together and discuss the significance of always listening to patient concerns. They discuss why a nurse must possess sound knowledge of disease processes and the drugs used to treat them. Matt also highlights to Chinyere the importance of providing patient education and information as an integral part of drug administration and how this can improve patient adherence/compliance with drug regimens. When Chinyere began the drug round with Matt, she thought she would learn about individual drugs and practise how to safely administer medication under supervision. She now realises that safe and effective drug administration is not just about giving the right drug to a patient, but also involves knowledge and understanding of the patient, disease processes and basic pharmacology.

This case study highlights that drug administration is not solely a mechanistic process (NMC, 2018). Safe and effective drug administration encompasses numerous dimensions, including effective communication, multidisciplinary teamwork, knowledge and understanding of pathophysiology, basic pharmacology and the overall patient's condition. Alongside these, nurses must use professional judgement and critical thinking skills, and base their decisions on sound evidence and knowledge.

This chapter is divided into three sections:

- understanding pharmacology;
- introducing medicines management;
- drug calculations.

The first section will focus on introductory pharmacology and its application to clinical practice. Two key concepts of pharmacology, pharmacokinetics and pharmacodynamics, will be explained and related to common drugs you may see in clinical practice. The second part will describe some of the processes involved in enabling you to safely and effectively administer medication under supervision in clinical practice. These include different routes of drug administration, the six rights of drug administration and understanding how drug errors can occur in clinical practice. Finally, the third part will provide a step-by-step guide to basic drug calculations relating to oral, intramuscular (IM) and subcutaneous medication.

Understanding pharmacology

What is pharmacology?

At its most basic level, pharmacology simply describes how drugs work in the body. Two concepts are key to understanding pharmacology:

- *Pharmacokinetics*: how the drug is treated as it moves through the body.
- *Pharmacodynamics*: how the drug affects the body.

Activity 8.1 Evidence-based practice and research

An asthmatic patient is diagnosed with high blood pressure (hypertension) and prescribed a *beta blocker* (to reduce high blood pressure). Following administration, they experience a severe asthma attack.

- Why did this occur?

An outline answer can be found at the end of the chapter.

Pharmacological knowledge is required at every stage of drug administration. Consider Activity 8.1 and how the administration of a beta blocker to an asthmatic patient can potentially lead to an asthma attack. All drugs have side effects, and understanding the disease, the drug and the patient condition means that you are able to safely assess, treat and monitor your patient for potential adverse reactions. Figure 8.1 outlines the pharmacological knowledge a nurse should understand before, during and after drug administration.

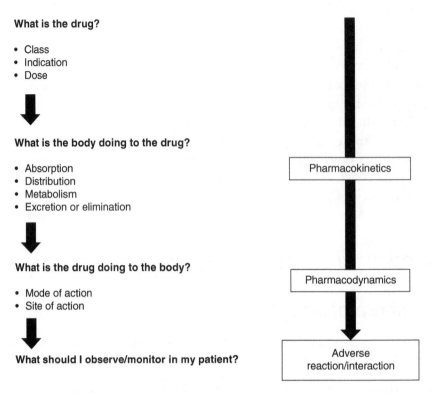

What is the drug?

- Class
- Indication
- Dose

What is the body doing to the drug?

- Absorption
- Distribution
- Metabolism
- Excretion or elimination

Pharmacokinetics

What is the drug doing to the body?

- Mode of action
- Site of action

Pharmacodynamics

What should I observe/monitor in my patient?

Adverse reaction/interaction

Figure 8.1 Pharmacological knowledge and drug adminstration

It is unrealistic to expect nurses to know every drug that is prescribed in minute detail. However, to safely administer any drug, a nurse should possess knowledge of all the information provided in Figure 8.1. Drug administration is a multidisciplinary procedure and as such if you lack the knowledge and understanding of how to administer a particular medication, you should always seek guidance first.

In clinical practice, pharmacists are available to provide expert information, advice and guidance on all matters relating to drug prescribing, dispensing, administration and monitoring. You will also come across the pharmaceutical reference guide: *British National Formulary* (BNF) in all clinical areas. Now available as a textbook, online and an app, it provides key information on prescribing, dispensing and administration of drugs.

All nurses should become familiar with navigating the BNF on a regular basis. It will provide you with up-to-date evidence-based information on drug indications, contra-indications, side effects and doses, alongside some basic pharmacology, drug overdoses and common interactions (Appendix 1). Complete Activity 8.2 to learn how to use the BNF.

Activity 8.2   Critical thinking

The BNF is updated twice a year (March and September). Use the most recent copy you can locate in the library to answer the following questions.

1.   What is the maximum daily dose of paracetamol for an adult?

2.   What is the recommended dose of aspirin for an adult diagnosed with cardiovascular disease (secondary prevention)?

3.   What are the most common or very common general side effects of the antihistamine drug chlorphenamine maleate?

4.   How many times a day should the proton pump inhibitor, omeprazole, be administered for a patient with a duodenal ulcer?

5.   Are nausea and vomiting common side effects of the antibiotic amoxicillin?

An outline answer can be found at the end of the chapter.

Pharmacokinetics

Once a drug is administered, it must move through the body to its intended site of action to produce an effect. How the body deals with a drug during its journey is known as pharmacokinetics and involves four distinct processes (known as ADME):

*   *Absorption*: how does the drug get into the body?
*   *Distribution*: how is the drug moved to its intended site of action?
*   *Metabolism*: how is the drug activated/inactivated?
*   *Excretion or elimination*: how will the drug be removed from the body?

Absorption deals with how a drug gets into the body and distribution is concerned with how a drug reaches its intended site of action. Metabolism will either activate or inactivate a drug and, finally, elimination is concerned with removing a drug from the body. Numerous individual, physical, biological and chemical factors can affect the ADME processes. Figure 8.2 summarises the four pharmacokinetic processes and some of the factors involved.

Absorption: how does the drug get into the body?

For a drug to produce a therapeutic response in an individual, it must reach its intended site of action at the right concentration. Absorption describes the movement of a drug from its site of administration across various biological membranes to the systemic circulation.

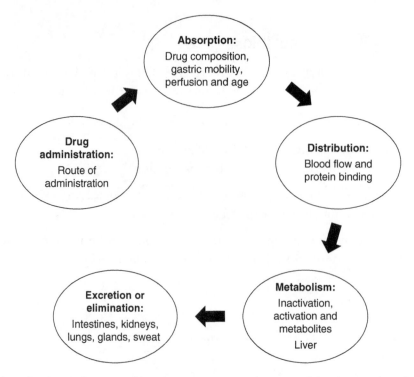

Figure 8.2   The four pharmacokinetic processes and some of the factors involved

Absorption in the gastrointestinal tract

In clinical practice you mainly witness drugs being administered via the oral route. Absorption of oral drugs mainly occurs in the small intestine. Drug absorption in the stomach is limited due to its thick mucus layer and highly acidic environment (pH 1–2) (Nair and Peate, 2013). The absorptive capacity of the small intestine is increased by the presence of villi and the permeability of thinner cell membranes, and is highly vascularised compared to the stomach.

First pass metabolism

Before a drug can be distributed to the systemic circulation and its intended site of action, oral drugs absorbed from the small intestine will travel to the liver. Approximately 80 per cent of all drugs that enter the liver at this point are metabolised and no longer active – that is, they cannot produce an effect. This is known as first pass metabolism and helps us to understand why some drugs cannot be administered via the oral route or must be given in higher doses. Both GTN (a potent vasodilator used in the treatment of angina) and fentanyl (opioid analgesic) are subject to extensive hepatic first pass metabolism and therefore have no therapeutic benefit when administered vial the oral route.

Only oral drugs are subject to the first pass effect. Drugs administered via the intra-muscular (IM), subcutaneous (SC) and intravenous (IV) route will directly enter the systemic circulation and avoid first pass metabolism in the liver. Figure 8.3 outlines the route of oral and intravenous drugs to the systemic circulation.

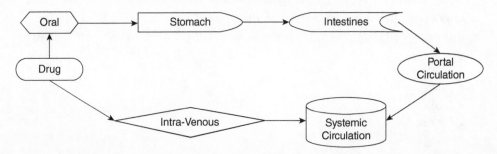

Figure 8.3 The simple route of delivery of oral and IV drug routes to the systemic circulation

Factors affecting drug absorption

Multiple factors can affect drug absorption and include lipid (fat) solubil-ity of a drug, gastric emptying and perfusion, presence of food or drugs in the gastro-intestinal system (GIT) and drug formulation. Some of the major factors influencing drug absorption are:

- lipid solubility;
- drug composition, formulation and size;
- route of administration;
- GIT motility and perfusion;
- acidic stomach environment;
- presence of food or drugs in GIT;
- food–drug interactions;
- presence of antacids in the GIT;
- first pass metabolism.

Gastric emptying, perfusion and the presence of food

Both reduced and accelerated gastric motility can affect the rate and degree of drug absorption. For example, diarrhoea and vomiting will accelerate gastric emptying and potentially reduce the effectiveness of medication administered orally. Other factors that affect peristalsis, such as older age, reduced mobility and the presence of food or certain drugs in the GIT, can affect absorption of some drugs. The absorption of Flucloxacillin, for example, is impaired by the presence of food in the stomach and should be taken on an empty stomach or at least two hours before food.

Drug formulation

Activity 8.3   Critical thinking

In clinical practice, drugs are available in multiple formulations which can affect both the rate and degree of absorption from the GIT. What do the following drug abbreviations indicate in relation to the absorption of a drug?

- LA
- MR
- SR
- EC

An outline answer can be found at the end of the chapter.

Activity 8.3 highlights how important it is for you to understand the formulation of the drug being administered. Many drugs are formulated to be absorbed slowly or at a controlled rate from the GIT and, as a result, administered less frequently. Other drugs are coated or wrapped in a polymer layer (similar to an M&M crispy outer coating) which prevents or delays absorption in the GIT. Aspirin is a good example of an enteric-coated drug designed to withstand the acidic stomach environment, allowing for absorption in the small intestine and preventing gastric irritation. Manipulating or altering formulations of drugs prior to administration can lead to adverse and potentially toxic or sub- therapeutic effects in patients.

Distribution: how is the drug moved to its intended site of action?

Once a drug is absorbed, it must then reach its intended site of action to produce an effect. Distribution simply describes the movement of a drug through the circulatory system to its intended site of action in the body. The distribution of drugs around the body is both unequal and uniform principally due to blood flow. Areas of the body which receive a high blood flow (and are well perfused), such as the heart, lungs and brain will receive the drug at a faster rate and in higher concentration than areas less well perfused, such as adipose tissue and bone.

Plasma protein binding

All drugs in the circulatory system will to some degree bind to plasma proteins (albumin) to prevent immediate excretion from the body. A drug bound to plasma proteins is in effect inactive. They are unable to diffuse from the circulatory system into tissues and cannot either exert an effect or be excreted. Only the 'unbound' drug – that is, not attached to plasma proteins – can move from the circulatory system into tissues and produce an effect. Figure 8.4 outlines the process of plasma protein binding.

The process of protein binding is in a constant flux, where bound drugs are automatically released as the unbound drug is metabolised and excreted. In normal health, the ratio between the bound and unbound drug in the body remains constant. Drugs attached to plasma proteins in the circulatory system are inactive – that is, unable to exert an effect, unable to diffuse into tissues and cannot be metabolised or excreted.

Plasma protein binding is not clinically significant. However, it may be of clinical consequence in particular disease states, such as liver cirrhosis or acute infection, or when two highly protein-bound drugs are co-administered to a patient. The case study below provides an example of the consequences of co-administration of two highly protein bound drugs.

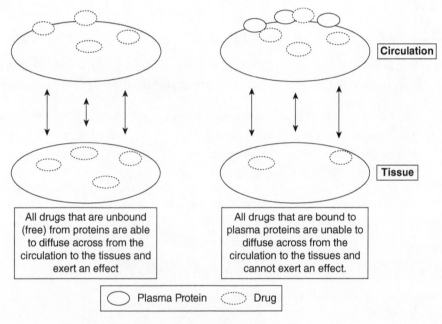

Figure 8.4 The process of plasma protein binding

Case study: Cheng

Cheng has been taking Warfarin for over five years for atrial fibrillation (Irregular heart rate). During a period of particularly bad weather and snowfall, he slips over and sprains his ankle. Cheng decides not to visit his GP and manages the pain by taking regular aspirin. Over the next couple of weeks while taking the aspirin and warfarin, Cheng has suffered from frequent nose bleeds and notices small bruises over his body.

In the case study above, Cheng has decided to self-administer aspirin while taking warfarin. Both of these drugs are highly protein bound and aspirin will compete with warfarin for circulating proteins. Aspirin is more competitive than warfarin for protein-binding sites, however, and will dislodge warfarin from their proteins, resulting in more unbound warfarin able to exert an effect. Cheng's symptoms of frequent nose bleeds and bruising are a direct result of increasing amounts of warfarin in his circulation and potentially can lead to increased risk of haemorrhage.

Activity 8.4 below will help you to understand protein binding and the consequences of co-administering two highly bound drugs in more detail. It should be pointed out that in some clinical situations, co-administration of two highly bound drugs may be appropriate. Drug administration should be both patient-centred and multidisciplinary in its approach. Fundamental to this would be patient education, careful monitoring, and involvement of nurses, pharmacists and doctors to mitigate adverse events.

Activity 8.4   Critical thinking

1. Warfarin is highly protein bound: 97 per cent. Which of the following drugs may potentially result in adverse events if co-administered with Warfarin?

    - Carbamazepine 75 per cent protein bound.
    - Digoxin 25 per cent protein bound.
    - Lithium 0 per cent protein bound.
    - Aspirin 90 per cent protein bound.

2. Consider the co-prescription of warfarin and sodium valproate to a patient.

    - What could be the consequences for the patient and why?

Use the BNF (Appendix 1) to inform your answer to this question.

An outline answer can be found at the end of the chapter.

Blood brain barrier

Case study: Jack

Jack is 16 years old and has developed the symptoms of hay fever, especially during the summer months. He is about to start his final year exams and visits his local chemist to buy some antihistamine drugs. The pharmacist advises Jack to take Cetirizine rather than chlorpheniramine to prevent the side effect of drowsiness while he is revising.

The brain protects itself from potentially harmful substances in the circulatory system, including drugs, with a highly selective protective layer of endothelial cells, held together tightly, called the blood brain barrier (BBB). To some degree, it is similar to a firewall used in computer systems. The BBB will only allow small lipid (fat) soluble and non-protein bound drugs to diffuse through. Examples of this include anaesthetic agents, antidepressants, hypnotic drugs and alcohol.

In the case study above, both chlorpheniramine and Cetirizine are lipophilic (fat-soluble) drugs and able to cross the blood brain barrier. However, cetirizine is a larger molecule and not as lipophilic as chlorpheniramine and therefore does not cross the BBB to the same degree, reducing the side effect of drowsiness.

Metabolism: how is a drug inactivated or activated?

Once a drug has reached its intended site of action and produced an effect, it needs to be eliminated from the body. If drugs were not metabolised and excreted, they would remain in the body, continually exerting an effect and potentially creating adverse reactions. Metabolism is the first stage in this process and predominantly occurs in the liver, and to a much smaller extent the plasma, GIT and lungs.

We typically assume that the liver only inactivates drugs ready for excretion. However, this is not strictly true. The liver will also chemically convert some drugs from an inactive to active form in the body, known as prodrugs. Examples of prodrugs include Levodopa, Enalapril and Ramipril.

In order to be excreted, drugs need to be in a hydrophilic (water) soluble form. This is one of the main functions of the liver: metabolism chemically alters a drug from an active lipophilic (fat) soluble state to a hydrophilic (water) inactive form ready for excretion. This is known as biotransformation and the altered final drug is now formed of metabolites. Very few drugs are able to be excreted without first undergoing metabolism.

This process is divided into two phases: phase 1 and phase 2. It is important to understand that these are not necessarily sequential, as some drugs will undergo one phase only and some both phases. A large family of enzymes in the liver called cytochrome P450 enzymes are important in the metabolism of drugs.

Phase 1 metabolism Cytochrome P450 enzymes will chemically alter the drug to a more water-soluble form mainly through the process of oxidation (adding oxygen) and, to a lesser extent, reduction (adding hydrogen) and hydrolysis (adding water).

Phase 2 metabolism This involves the addition of larger endogenous substances to a drug through the process of conjugation. Conjugation is an important chemical process that further increases the water solubility of a drug alongside inactivating it ready for excretion.

Enzyme induction and inhibition

The cytochrome P450 family of enzymes are responsible for metabolising up to 75 per cent of all drugs and each group can metabolise multiple drugs. When certain drugs or foods are metabolised by the same group of P450 enzymes, clinically significant drug–drug or food–drug interactions can occur through enzyme induction and inhibition. Appendix 1 of the BNF provides a useful list of potential drug interactions.

Factors affecting metabolism

Activity 8.5 is designed to help you to explore and think of the factors that affect drug metabolism.

Activity 8.5   Critical thinking

Make a list of some of the physiological and pathological factors that you think can affect drug metabolism.

An outline answer can be found at the end of the chapter.

As you have learnt, metabolism is an important pharmacokinetic principle for both activation and inactivation and subsequent elimination of drugs. Changes to liver function can potentially lead to toxic adverse effects and drug doses are commonly reduced to mitigate these risks (BNF provides details on this). Completing Activity 8.6 can help you understand why some drugs are contraindicated or doses reduced in patients in some clinical conditions.

Excretion or elimination: how the drug will be removed from the body

Activity 8.6 is designed to help you identify the different ways in which drugs are excreted from the human body.

Activity 8.6   Evidence-based practice and research

Drug excretion is the removal of a drug from the body. Make a list of all the routes of drug excretion from the body.

An outline answer can be found at the end of the chapter.

Activity 8.6 highlights the multiple routes of drug excretion from the body. Most of the routes you will have identified only play a minor role in drug excretion. By far the most important organ for drug excretion is urine via the kidneys. Drugs are moved from plasma through three renal mechanisms: glomular filtration, active tubular secretion and active tubular reabsorption. Figure 8.5 outlines some of the processes involved.

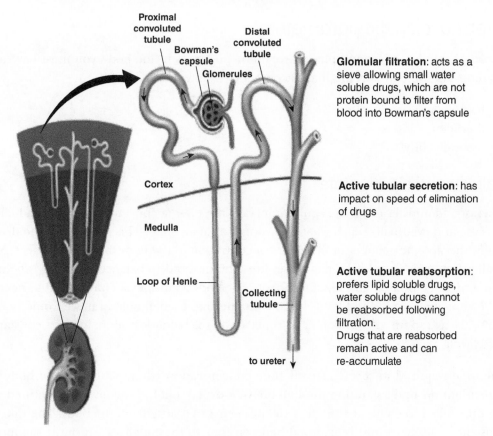

Glomular filtration: acts as a sieve allowing small water soluble drugs, which are not protein bound to filter from blood into Bowman's capsule

Active tubular secretion: has impact on speed of elimination of drugs

Active tubular reabsorption: prefers lipid soluble drugs, water soluble drugs cannot be reabsorbed following filtration.
Drugs that are reabsorbed remain active and can re-accumulate

Figure 8.5 Some of the processes involved in renal excretion

Factors affecting renal excretion

Many factors can affect drug excretion, including perfusion, renal blood flow, cardiac failure, renal disease and the ageing process. The administration of drugs to individuals with reduced renal function can potentially cause adverse effects, including toxicity. Careful assessment and monitoring by nurses is essential to prevent this. Activity 8.7 is designed to help you think about assessment when considering drug administration to a patient.

Activity 8.7   Critical thinking

In clinical practice, you may come across many different options for drug dosing in renal impairment. Most commonly, the dose will be reduced or the drug stopped if possible. What other options are available?

An outline answer can be found at the end of the chapter.

The next section focuses on helping you to understand pharmacokinetic processes. Examples are provided to help you better understand this concept.

Pharmacokinetic parameters

In order to fully understand pharmacokinetic processes in the body, you must have an awareness of some important pharmacokinetic parameters:

- half-life and steady state;
- therapeutic index;
- bioavailability.

Half-life and steady state

When we administer drugs at regular intervals, the plasma concentration will gradually increase and eventually reach what is known as a steady state. This means that the drug is now therapeutic – that is, at the right concentration in the body to exert an effect. An equilibrium is achieved if regular doses are administered to balance out what is being removed (metabolised and excreted) from the body. Consider a container that needs to be kept at a certain fluid level. If the container has a small hole in it, we would need to regularly 'top up' the container to replace what is being lost to maintain a constant fluid level.

The time required to reach a steady state concentration (therapeutic) in the body is dependent on understanding the half-life of a drug. Half-life is commonly defined as the time taken to eliminate one half (50 per cent) of a drug from the body. The rate is constant in all drugs and is achieved between four to five half-lives. Warfarin (an anti-coagulant) is a good example of a drug with a long half-life and the case study below outlines how this can effect its administration and monitoring.

Clinical example

Warfarin has a relatively long half-life of approximately 40 hours. In practical terms, this means it would take up to 48 hours after initial administration to produce a therapeutic effect. Warfarin is usually administered once a day due to its long half-life. The long half-life also means it may take up to five days to completely remove the drug from the body. This is an important concept if we are considering prescribing and administering a drug that may potentially clinically interact with Warfarin.

In clinical practice, to maintain a steady state, drugs with a short half-life will need to be administered more frequently or as a continuous infusion. Whereas drugs with a longer half-life can be administered less frequently, in some cases once a day as per our

---

example of Warfarin above. If a steady state needs to be achieved quickly, as in an acute infection such as meningitis, the blood plasma can be 'loaded' with antibiotics with an initial larger dose prior to regular dosing with the aim or reaching a steady state more quickly. It is vital that nurses understand the half-lives of the drugs they are administering, as it will determine the frequency of drug administration, affect how some drugs are administered and be useful regarding potential drug interactions.

Therapeutic index

Clinical example

A patient with meningitis is treated with high-dose Penicillin and Gentamycin. The plasma concentration levels of Gentamycin are monitored frequently but not the Penicillin. Why?

A therapeutic index is a clinically relevant factor which describes the range between the minimum effective dose and the minimum toxic dose of a drug. In the clinical example above, gentamycin has a narrow therapeutic index, meaning the margin between the drug being therapeutic and toxic is small. If the drug concentration levels are not carefully monitored, there is a risk of gentamycin becoming sub-therapeutic and essentially ineffective or toxic and producing adverse effects. Conversely, Penicillin has a large therapeutic index and so does not require drug monitoring.

In clinical practice, you will see drugs with a narrow therapeutic index being carefully monitored with regular blood tests. Dosages of the drug will then be titrated, depending on an individual patient's plasma concentration of the drug. As you can see, it is imperative that nurses know which drugs have a narrow therapeutic index to safely administer them. Common drugs with a narrow therapeutic index are Warfarin, digoxin, theophylline, vancomycin, gentamycin, lithium and cyclosporine.

Bioavailability

Bioavailability is an important pharmacokinetic principle and refers to the total amount of unchanged drug – that is, able to produce an effect – that reaches the intended site of action in the body from its site of administration. Multiple factors can influence the bioavailability of a drug, including first pass metabolism, route of administration, gastric acid, digestive enzymes and the presence of food or other drugs in the stomach. For example, consider why Insulin and Heparin are not administered via the oral route. This is because the bioavailability of Heparin and Insulin is vastly reduced by the presence of digestive enzymes in the stomach which destroy the drugs.

Individual factors affecting the pharmacokinetic process

Multiple individual factors can affect every aspect of the pharmacokinetic process when administering drugs. In contemporary nursing, our patient age profile is ever increasing. Older patients are more commonly at risk of drug-related adverse effects, which can potentially be detrimental to their health. Individual factors that can affect the pharmacokinetic process include gender, genetics, tolerance, weight, environmental factors, and pathological and physiological variables.

Pharmacodynamics

When we take an antihistamine drug to treat the symptoms of hay fever, for example, how does the drug know where to exert its effect in the body to reduce the symptoms? Understanding pharmacodynamics explains how drugs such as antihistamines work in our body to treat both the symptoms of hay fever and how side effects may occur.

Pharmacodynamics is most commonly defined as 'what the drug does to the body'. At a basic level, this involves the action of the drug at different sites in the body, its effect and any adverse effects it may cause. To produce an effect, a drug must bind with a specific site in the body. Most target sites for drug interaction in the body are proteins and involve four main types:

- receptors;
- ion channels;
- enzyme interaction;
- carrier/transport mechanisms.

Drugs and receptors

There are multiple receptor sites in the body which in normal health interact with endogenous ligands (chemicals) to maintain homeostasis. The vast majority of drugs interact and bind to receptors to either produce a response (agonist) or block a response (antagonist). In order to block or produce an effect, the drug must be structurally compatible with the relevant receptor site. The analogy of a lock and key is often used to explain this process: the right key (drug) must fit the right lock (receptor) to be effective. In this analogy, a natural ligand binding to a receptor would be equivalent to the correct key fitting a lock to produce an effect – in this case, opening the door. Following from this, an agonist can mimic a natural ligand to produce an effect in the same way that you can potentially open a door by picking the lock with a pin. Finally, it is also possible for an antagonist to bind to but not produce an effect. This is comparable to putting the wrong key into a locked door: it might fit the hole if it is close to the shape of the correct key but won't have the effect of opening the door.

We have multiple receptor sites in our bodies. Different drugs will work at many different receptor sites. When we learn about groups of drugs, understanding the class of the drug and the function of the relevant receptor will enable us to understand its mode of action in more detail. For example:

- Salbutamol is a β_2- adrenergic agonist used to treat asthma . We can see from this that it acts on β_2 receptors in the lungs to produce an effect (agonist) – in this case, bronchodilation.
- Let's return to our earlier example of antihistamines used to treat hay fever. Antihistamines belong to a class of drugs called histamine H_1 receptor antagonists. We can conclude from this that antihistamines antagonise (block) the effect of histamine release at the histamine H_1 receptor, reducing the inflammatory response. In fact, groups of drugs with the prefix 'blocker' or 'anti' at the beginning are always antagonists.

We can take this slightly further and gain information on the some of the potential side effects of a drug when we understand its class and mode of action. For example, as we have learnt, antihistamines work by blocking histamine H_1 receptors, reducing the inflammatory response but can also cause drowsiness as a side effect. This is because receptors located in our bodies are not found in only one location and drugs are not always specific for one receptor site.

Antihistamines will work on both peripheral and central histamine receptor sites, and will to some degree cross the blood brain barrier. The central actions of antihistamines on histamine receptors in the brain can result in drowsiness.

Drugs and ion channels

Numerous drugs will work on ion channels to antagonise (block) a response. Ion channels are formed of proteins found in cell membranes and will selectively allow the passage of ions such as potassium and sodium in and out of a cell to produce a physiological response in the body. Figure 8.6 outlines how ion channels work in the body. The two most common types of ion channels are:

1. Voltage-gated ion channels: ion channels activated by changes in a membrane potential.
2. Ligand-gated ion channels: endogenous ligands bind to the channel protein.

Two types of drugs will act at ion channels: channel blockers and channel modulators. Channel blockers bind to ion channels and block the transport of ions through to the cell, and channel modulators will bind to a receptor site within the ion channel and change the permeability of the membrane.

Examples of ion channel drugs

- Lidocaine can be used as a local anaesthetic to block peripheral pain signals, allowing for minor surgery and other surgical interventions such as suturing. Lidocaine will reversibly interrupt nerve conduction by preventing sodium ions from entering the nerve cell, thus blocking pain signals.
- Diltiazem will disrupt the movement of calcium through voltage-gated ion channels. The effect is reduced myocardial contractility and smooth muscle relaxation, both of which are useful in the treatment of hypertension.

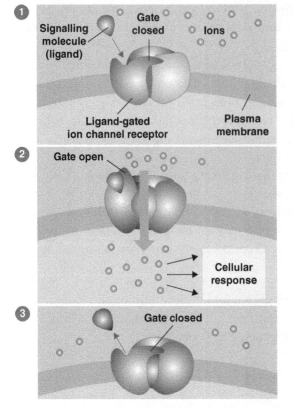

1: Both endogenous ligands and ions will circulate and attach to ion proteins found in the cell membrane

2: Once attached they will selectively allow transport through the cell to produce an effect

3: Once the ligand or ion is removed the gate will close and return to its resting potential.

Figure 8.6 Ions channels

Drugs and enzymes

Enzymes are proteins in the body that influence the rate and speed of chemical reactions in the body. These drugs are used in numerous diseases to either increase or decrease enzyme activity; most commonly, they inhibit.

Examples of enzyme-inhibiting drugs

- Ramipril, which is used in the treatment of hypertension and cardiac failure, inhibits the actions of the angiotensin-converting enzyme (ACE).
- Omeprazole comes from the class of drugs known as proton pump inhibitors (PPIs), because it reduces hydrochloric acid production by inhibiting the enzyme H^+/K^+-adenosine triphosphates (the proton pump), which is the final stage of acid production in the stomach.
- Aspirin is used to treat mild to moderate pain and possesses useful anti-inflammatory properties. Its mechanism of action is to block two cyclooxygenase enzymes known as COX-1 and COX-2. These are found throughout the body and produce prostaglandins which are implicated in producing pain and inflammation. Once COX-1 and COX-2 are blocked by aspirin, they are unable to produce the prostaglandins that cause the pain and inflammation.

Carrier/transport mechanisms and drugs

Some drugs are unable to enter the cell without essentially 'hitching a ride' from a carrier molecule. The drug will bind to the carrier protein in the cell wall and is then simply moved through the cell membrane into the cell. The most common examples of drugs that use carrier/transport mechanisms are selective serotonin reuptake inhibitors (SSRIs), Fluoxetine and Citalopram, used in the treatment of depression.

Introducing medicines management

In the United Kingdom (UK) medications are both the most common intervention and cause of harm to patients (NICE, 2015). Medication management is a significant nursing role and it is estimated that nurses spend up to 40 per cent of their clinical time administering drugs in the hospital setting. The second part of this chapter will focus on some of the factors involved in enabling you to safely and effectively administer medication under supervision in the clinical setting.

Routes of drug administration

As you will have observed in clinical practice, drugs can be administered by a variety of routes. The route of administration of a drug is a significant pharmacokinetic factor and to varying degrees will affect the therapeutic effect of the drug at its intended site of action.

Activity 8.8   Evidence-based practice and research

Make a list of all the different routes of drug administration you have seen in clinical practice.

An outline answer can be found at the end of the chapter.

Activity 8.8 illustrates the multiple routes of drug administration. By far the most common route of drug administration you will encounter in clinical practice is oral. Oral drug administration is convenient, practical, inexpensive and possibly the preferred option for most individuals.

Consider the administration of an antibiotic to a patient with an infection. It is possible to administer this drug via a variety of routes, including oral (PO), IM, IV and per rectum (PR). Multiple factors will influence and ultimately determine the most appropriate route of administration for the antibiotic, which effectively treats the infection. In this example, factors for consideration may include patient choice, bioavailability, drug characteristics and the overall condition of the patient.

Drug administration

Prescription drug charts

Although most hospital trusts will adopt their own version of an in-hospital prescription drug chart, the information provided is usually generic. Figure 8.7 shows the information provided on a prescription drug chart for regular prescriptions – that is, drugs taken at regular intervals and not as required or one-off (stat) medications. It is vital that nurses check each aspect of the drug chart for each individual prescription every time they administer a drug to a patient.

All information provided should be clear and legible, and if there any doubts regarding the legibility of any aspect of the prescription, it should be clarified with the prescriber and/or the pharmacist prior to administration. An explanation of each section is provided in Figure 8.7.

REGULAR PRESCRIPTIONS				Date						
DRUG (approved name)				Time						
Route	Dose	Start date	End date							
Signature		Pharmacy								
Special Instructions										

Figure 8.7   A sample drug chart for regular prescribed drugs

Drug (approved name): all drugs possess a trade (branded), generic (non-proprietary) and chemical name. The generic or non-proprietary name should be used on all drugs charts, unless otherwise specifically stated. This is to prevent potential drug errors in clinical practice – for example, the antibiotic Co-amoxiclav has the trade (branded) name Augmentin®. Both contain a penicillin combination and should not be administered to penicillin-sensitive patients. The BNF and/or the pharmacist can provide information on all recommended drug names.

Route: this should be clear and legible, and in capital letters to avoid ambiguity in drug administration. Only individual trust-approved abbreviations should be used to avoid misunderstandings, which may result in medication administration errors.

Dose: this should be clear and legible to the person administering the drug. Any ambiguity with the drug dose should be checked with the prescriber/BNF/pharmacist as appropriate. The unit of measure must be included for all drug doses. To limit the potential drug errors associated with the use of micrograms in clinical practice, it is usually written in full and not abbreviated.

Start and end date: all drugs prescribed should have a start date (the date the medication was originally prescribed, if possible) and an end date (when required). An end date is especially important with prescriptions of antibiotics, where a short course – for example, three or five days – is prescribed.

Signature: drugs should never be administered if a signature of the prescriber is not present on the drug chart. The original prescriber should be contacted to sign the drug chart before the drug is administered to the patient.

Pharmacy: all wards and departments in a hospital setting should have a named pharmacist who will visit at regular intervals during normal working hours. A part of their responsibility is to check all drug charts for accuracy and potential problems. Pharmacists usually write in green ink on drug charts and initial this box when they have checked them. They may add further information or amend a drug chart; again, this is usually written in green ink.

Special instructions: any special instructions related to the administration or monitoring of the drug that the prescriber or pharmacist feels the person administering the drug needs to know will be written here. For example, instructions on administering Flucloxacillin on an empty stomach or two hours before food may be written here.

Date: the date, including day, month and year must be clearly written in this section.

Time: some drug charts will have pre-printed timings, otherwise it should be the prescriber who clearly identifies the timings for administering the drug on the drug chart and not the person administering the medication.

Hospital e-prescribing and drug administration

Some National Health Service (NHS) trusts have adopted Hospital e-Prescribing and Drug Administration (HePMA) in recent years. There is some evidence that this system reduces drug errors in clinical practice by up to 50 per cent with high-risk medications, and is more cost-effective (DHSC, 2016).

All digital systems can be a challenge, and thorough training and on-going support is required for successful implementation. To date, the implementation of HePMA across the NHS is variable. Figures from November 2017 suggest that only 35 per cent of acute trusts and 12 per cent of mental health organisations have adopted the system (DHSC, 2016).

The six rights of drug administration

Safe and effective drug administration for patients requires a knowledgeable and competent nurse who appreciates the complexities of medicines management and pharmacology (NMC, 2018). A common approach advocated to improve safety and mitigate potential drug errors is the implementation of the six rights

(6Rs) of drug administration. The 6Rs should be applied to every single drug administration by a nurse. The 6Rs of drug administration are:

- right patient;
- right drug;
- right dose;
- right route;
- right time;
- right documentation.

Right patient

The medication must be administered to the correct patient. The hospital identification number and date of birth (DOB) should be cross-referenced with the drug chart and the patient identity wrist-band. Although we may ask the patient to state their name and DOB, this approach alone can lead to potential drug errors in a hospital setting. The patient may have cognitive impairment such as dementia or deafness, or there may be another patient with the same or similar name in the ward or department. Drug allergies should be confirmed at this stage, both verbally if appropriate and a record of allergies should be written on a drug chart and the patient provided with a red identification wrist- band if they have an allergy.

Right drug

Electronic prescribing has reduced some of the issues related to poor handwriting and legibility with drug prescriptions. If the prescription is handwritten, it should be clear and legible, and the generic name of the drug used in most cases. If there is any doubt on the part of the person administering the medication, they should not administer the drug and contact the prescriber and/or pharmacist. The name of the drug written on the drug chart should be checked against the label on the carton or bottle supplied.

Right dose

If you are unfamiliar with the drug and do not know the correct dosage range, this must be checked prior to administration using the BNF. You may need to calculate the actual dose of the medicine. Competence in drug calculations is a prerequisite for all drug administrations.

Right route

Is the route on the prescription appropriate and does it match the route of the drug available? Are there any specific instructions for the drug and is it available in different formulations? For example, should the drug be administered on an empty stomach or with food? Can the patient take the drug via the prescribed route?

Right time

All medications need to be administered at the correct time to ensure a therapeutic steady state of the drug in the body.

Right documentation

It is a professional and legal requirement that all prescription charts are signed *after* the drug is administered. Signing the drug chart before the drug is administered can lead to several issues – for example, the patient may refuse or forget to take the medication, and may for some other reason not be able to take the medication – for example, due to nausea or vomiting. Failure to sign a drug chart after administration of a drug can lead to potential drug errors, as another nurse may believe the drug has not been administered if it is not signed and then repeat the dose, leading to potential adverse effects. If you are unable to administer the drug for some reason, this must be documented on the drug chart.

Medication errors in clinical practice

A recent report, published in March 2018, estimated that 237 million drug errors occur at some point in the medication process in England per year and 66 million of these were clinically significant (Elliott, et al., 2018). Nurses are frequently cited as the last line of defence in preventing a drug error as they are usually at the final stage of the medicines management process – drug administration. However, drug errors are possible at every stage of the medicines management process: prescribing, dispensing, administration and monitoring.

Defining drug errors

Defining drug errors can be difficult and as a consequence has to some degree led to an underreporting in clinical practice. A drug error can be simply defined as a *preventable event that may lead to inappropriate medication use or patient harm* (Elliott et al., 2018, p4). Consider the definition of a drug error presented above and complete Activity 8.9.

Activity 8.9   Critical thinking

Which of the following would you consider a drug error?

1.   A patient missed a dose of antibiotics due to being away from the ward.

2.   A dose of antibiotics is delayed by 50 minutes.

3.   The nurse omitted the 00:00hr antibiotic as the patient was asleep.

An outline answer can be found at the end of the chapter.

We can apply some of the pharmacological processes we have discussed in this chapter to help us understand why knowledge of pharmacology is so important for nurses. For example, the importance of maintaining a therapeutic drug concentration (steady state) is dependent on regular drug administration at defined intervals. Understanding the half-life off a drug means that we know there are specific timings in relation to drug administration to remain therapeutic. The patient in all these questions could potentially have a serious infection. Missing or delaying one dose of antibiotics may seem trivial, but it could potentially lead to deterioration and life-threatening sepsis, depending on the clinical condition of the patient.

Causes of drug errors

Case study: Joe

Joe qualified six months ago and is working on a busy medical ward and allocated eight patients due to the ward being short-staffed today. He is running late with his workload and begins the lunchtime medication round late. During the medication round, he is interrupted by a colleague, a patient who wants to use the toilet and the porter with the lunchtime food trolley. Two of the drugs he needs to administer are not available on the drug trolley and he has to stop the drug round to obtain these from the treatment room. Once Joe finishes the drug round, he realises he has administered the wrong drug to a patient.

What factors do you think led to Joe's drug error?

As you can see from the case study, multiple factors can contribute to drug errors in clinical practice. Joe is newly qualified and inexperienced, and may be lacking in confidence. The ward is short-staffed, he has been allocated more patients than usual and running late with the lunchtime drug round. He may be stressed and anxious about his workload and, due to time limits, not concentrating and rushing to finish the drug round. During the drug round Joe is interrupted numerous times. Interruptions during drug rounds are considered to be one of the most important factors contributing to drug errors in clinical practice. Some of the factors that may contribute to drug errors in clinical practice can be attributable to working conditions, which include shortage of staff, poor skill mix, slow pharmacy delivery, a high workload, a busy ward, long or complex medication rounds, a long working day and a lack of patient acuity. Another factor is lack of knowledge, including knowledge of the drug disease status of the patient. The nurse's level of experience is important: inexperienced staff can easily lead to a general lack of confidence, or even to a miscalculation of drugs. There are also a number of external factors that could include interruptions during the drug round, unclear packaging of medication, tiredness or stress, poor communication skills, lack of attention to detail, complacency and prescription illegibility.

Drug calculations

The final part of this chapter provides a step-by-step guide to understanding basic drug calculations commonly encountered in clinical practice. The following calculations will be covered:

- Converting metric units.
- Calculating the dose required (tablets and capsules).
- Calculating drug volumes (tablets, capsules and injections).
- Calculating doses according to body weight.
- Calculating the maximum daily amount of a drug a patient can receive in a 24-hour period (tablets and capsules).

All answers to the exercises are provided at the end of the chapter.

Converting metric units

All drug doses and volumes are calculated using the International System of Units, abbreviated to SI units. When drug calculations are performed, the same unit of measurement must be used in the calculation, so knowledge of converting SI units is a prerequisite. Table 8.1 outlines the most common SI units you will come across in nursing.

Units of weight	
1 kilogram (kg)	= 1000 grams (g)
1 gram (g)	= 1000 milligrams (mg)
1 milligram (mg)	= 1000 micrograms (mcg)
Units of volume	
1 litre (l)	= 1000 millilitres (ml)

Table 8.1   Common SI units of weights and volumes

In order to administer the correct dose of a drug, we frequently need to convert the weight or volume first. For example:

- mcg ↔ mg or mg ↔ mcg
- mg ↔ g or g ↔ mg

Converting from a bigger to a smaller unit

To calculate from a *bigger unit to a smaller unit* – for example, grams (g) to milligrams (mg), we multiply by 1000. Essentially, we move the decimal point three points to the right.

Example

You are required to convert 5 grams (g) to milligrams (mg). To complete this, multiply 5 by 1000, which gives you 5000mg.

Exercise 1

1. Convert 2g to mg.

2. Convert 57g to mg.

3. Convert 124mg to mcg.

4. Convert 674 mg to mcg.

5. Convert 1.2g to mg.

6. Convert 8.4g to mg.

7. Convert 0.05mg to mcg.

8. Convert 62.5mg to mcg.

Converting from a smaller to a bigger unit

To calculate from a *smaller to bigger unit* – for example, micrograms (mcg) to milligram (mg) – we divide by 1000. Essentially, we move the decimal point three points to the left.

Example

You need to find out how many grams are in 1250mg. You do this by dividing 1250 by 1000 to give you 1.25g.

Exercise 2

1. Convert 43mcg to mg.

2. Convert 357mcg to mg.

3. Convert 253mg to g.

4. Convert 342mg to g.

5. Convert 1000mg to g.

6. Convert 1500mg to g.

7. Convert 500mcg to mg.

8. Convert 874mcg to mg.

Calculating the dose required (tablets and capsules)

Most drugs are prescribed according to the dose range or strength available – for example, a patient is prescribed 50mg Tramadol and the dose or strength available is 50mg. However, sometimes the dose prescribed does not match the strength of the tablet or capsule available. In this instance, you are required to calculate the amount of tablets or capsules required for the dose prescribed.

Calculating the dose required involves using a simple formula:

$$\text{Dose required} = \frac{\text{Amount prescribed}}{\text{Amount in each tablet or capsule available}}$$

Example

A patient is prescribed 100 microgram (mcg) of Levothyroxine and the strength of the tablets available is 25mcg. How many tablets are required?

Using the above formula:

$$\frac{100}{25} = 4$$

4 tablets are required for this dose.

Remember that the units must always be the same when calculating the dose required and it is often easier to convert them before you use the formula.

Example

A patient is prescribed 2g of Amoxicillin. The dose available is 500mg capsules. How many capsules are required for this dose?

Step 1

Convert the g → mg first

$2 \times 1000 = 2000$mg

Step 2

Now use the formula:

$$\frac{2000}{500} = 4$$

4 capsules are required for this dose.

Exercise 3

1. A patient is prescribed 150mg of Ranitidine and the strength of the tablets available is 75mg. How many tablets are required?

2. A patient is prescribed 750mg of Ciprofloxacillin and the strength of the tablets available is 250mg. How many tablets are required?

3. A patient is prescribed 400mg of Trimethoprim and the strength of the tablets is 200mg. How many tablets are required?

4. A patient is prescribed 2.5g of Flucloxacillin and the strength of the capsules available is 500mg. How many capsules are required?

5. A patient is prescribed 1g of Amoxicillin. The stock dose is 500mg tablets. How many tablets will you administer?

Calculating drug volumes

The following formulas can be used to calculate the volume of the drug to be given.

$$\text{Volume required} = \frac{\text{what you want}}{\text{what you've got}} \times \text{volume available}$$

or

$$\frac{\text{Dose prescribed}}{\text{dose available}} \times \text{volume of solution}$$

or

NHS formula: (need, have and solution)

$$\frac{\text{need}}{\text{have}} \times \text{solution}$$

Example 1

Paracetamol is available as 25mg in 5ml and we need to give the patient 50mg. How many ml would you draw up? Using the formulas above:

$$\frac{50}{25} \times 5 = 10$$

So you are required to administer 10ml of paracetamol.

Example 2

You can also use a worked method for this type of question, for example:

A patient is prescribed 2.5mg of a drug and the concentration available is 10mg/10ml. How many ml would you draw up?

So:

10mg = 10ml

5mg = 5ml

2.5mg = 2.5ml

So you would draw up 2.5ml.

Exercise 4

1. Drug available as 10mg/2ml: prescription is for 20mg. How many ml will you draw up?

2. Drug available as 5mg/5ml: prescription is for 2.5mg. How many ml would you draw up?

3. Drug available as 2.5mg/10ml: prescription is for 7.5mg. How many ml would you draw up?

4. Drug available as 25mg/ml, how many mg are there in 5ml?

5. Drug available as 5mg/ml, how many mg are there in 15ml?

6. The dose required is 25mg. The concentration available is 10mg/5ml. How many ml would you draw up?

7. The dose required is 75mg. The concentration available is 15mg/3ml. How may ml should you administer?

Doses according to body weight

More frequently, the dose required is based on the patient's body weight. Calculating the dose required according to body weight uses a simple formula:

Total dose required = dose per kg × patient's weight

Example 1

The dose required is 3mg/kg and the patient weighs 68kg.

This means that for every kg of the patient's weight, you are required to administer 3mg of the drug.

So, multiply 68 by 3, which gives you 204mg.

Therefore, the patient requires a total dose of 204mg.

Example 2

A patient is prescribed 100mg/kg and weighs 50kg. What is the total dose in grams?

$100 \times 50 = 5000mg$

However, we are required to provide the answer in grams.

We must convert the units once we have worked out the dose in milligrams (mg):

$$\frac{5000}{1000} = 5$$

So the answer is 5g.

Remember the rule: same units before starting the calculation.

Exercise 5

1. The dose required is 11mg/kg and the patient weighs 77kg. What is the total dose in mg?

2. The dose required is 0.5mg/kg and the patient weighs 55kg. What is the total dose in mg?

3. The dose required is 2.5mg/kg and the patient weighs 106kg.What is the total dose in mg?

4. The dose required is 2mcg/kg and the patient weighs 54kg. What is the total dose in mcg?

5. The dose required is 50mg/kg and the patient weighs 80kg. What is the total dose in grams?

6. The dose required is 100mg/kg and the patient weighs 65kg. What is the total dose in grams?

Maximum daily amount of tablets or capsules in a 24-hour period

All drugs have a maximum prescribed number of tablets or capsules that can be administered in a 24-hour period and the BNF will provide this information for most medications. For example, the dose of paracetamol in the BNF is 0.5g–1g every 4–6 hours to a maximum dose of 4g daily. Therefore, as nurses, we are required to work out how many tablets or capsules a patient can receive in a 24-hour period. This is of particular importance when administering as required or PRN medication doses.

Example

The maximum daily amount of paracetamol is 4g in 24 hours. How many 500mg tablets can the patient receive in a 24-hour period?

Step 1

Convert grams → mg

4 x 1000 = 4000

Step 2

Divide by the concentration of the tablet:

$$\frac{4000}{500} = 8$$

So the patient can receive a total of 8 tablets in a 24-hour period.

Exercise 6

1. The maximum daily amount of a drug is 6g. How many 500mg tablets can the patient receive?

2. The maximum daily amount of a drug is 240mg. How many 30mg tablets can the patient receive?

3. The maximum daily amount of a drug is 600mg. How many 150mg tablets can the patient receive?

Chapter summary

This chapter has provided you with an overview of some of the factors involved in safe and effective drug administration in clinical practice. It is vital that nurses have a thorough understanding of pharmacology, disease processes, the patient condition and the drug every time they administer medication.

The NMC Standards for Pre-registration Nursing Education generic competencies were outlined in relation to Medicines Management Essential Skill Cluster. These generic competencies and subsequent scenario and activities emphasise the need for the ability to calculate drugs, numeracy, up-to-date knowledge and evidence to assess, plan, deliver and evaluate care, communicate findings, affect change, and promote health and best practice.

This was achieved by addressing current and up-to-date referenced evidence and the basic principles of pharmacokinetics and pharmacodynamics. The case studies allowed the issue of safety, patient education, communication and informed consent to be demonstrated. The subject of medication errors was also addressed and it was seen that this event could lead to potential and actual patient harm.

The need for the nurse to administer safe patient-centred care, legal and ethical evidence-based decision-making, in addition to acknowledging the complexity of clinical decision-making was demonstrated. Knowing when specialist knowledge and intervention are required have also been addressed. It was seen that this knowledge is essential for high quality and the best possible outcomes of care in relation to pharmacology and medicines management.

Activities: Brief outline answers

Activity 8.1   Evidence-based practice and research (p173)

Some beta blockers (Propranolol) are non-selective – that is, they will also block receptors located in the lungs, causing bronchoconstriction. For some susceptible patients with asthma, this can precipitate an asthma attack. More modern beta blockers are now available that are selective for receptors in the heart and not the lungs, and will not cause this adverse effect.

Activity 8.2   Critical thinking (p175)

1.   4g per day.

2.   75mg daily.

3.   Blurred vision, dry mouth and drowsiness.

4.   By mouth: 20mg once a day for four weeks and increased to 40mg daily in severe or recurrent cases.

5.   Yes, nausea and vomiting are common or very common side effects.

Activity 8.3   Critical thinking (p178)

LA: Long acting

MR: Modified release

SR: Slow release

EC: Enteric coated

Activity 8.4   Critical thinking (p180)

1.   All the drugs with high protein binding can potentially cause adverse events if co-administered. In this case, both Carbamazepine and Aspirin are likely to lead to an increased risk of adverse events and would need to be carefully monitored.

2.   Both of these drugs are highly protein-bound (>90 per cent) and co-administration can lead to competition at protein-binding sites, similar to the example of aspirin in the main text. According to Appendix 1 in the BNF, this can be clinically significant and lead to a rapid rise in a patient's INR, resulting in increased risk of haemorrhaging.

Activity 8.5   Critical thinking (p182)

Factors affecting drug metabolism include genetic variations, increasing age, liver disease which results in the destruction of hepatocytes such as cirrhosis, and conditions such as heart failure and shock which can cause reduced hepatic blood flow.

Activity 8.6   Evidence-based practice and research (p182)

Routes of drug elimination or excretion include the kidneys, bile, lungs, breast milk, perspiration, saliva and tears.

Activity 8.7   Critical thinking (p183)

Other options for drug administration in renal failure include changing the drug to one that is not excreted via the kidneys, increasing the dosing intervals between the drugs, monitoring the drug plasma concentration at a more regular interval if possible and monitoring the patient's renal function more frequently.

Activity 8.8   Evidence-based practice and research (p189)

Different routes of drug administration:

Intravenous (IV), intramuscular (IM), subcutaneous (SC), sublingual or buccal, inhalation, rectal (PR), oral (PO), transdermal (topical) and per vagina (PV).

Activity 8.9   Critical thinking (p193)

Options 2 and 3 can be considered a drug error.

Drug calculation exercises: Answers

Exercise 1

1. 2000mg
2. 57000mg
3. 124000mcg
4. 674000mcg
5. 1200mg
6. 8400mg
7. 50mcg
8. 62500mcg

Exercise 2

1. 0.043mg
2. 0.357mg
3. 0.253g
4. 0.342g
5. 1g
6. 1.5g
7. 0.5mg
8. 0.874mg

Exercise 3

1. 2 tablets
2. 3 tablets
3. 2 tablets
4. 5 capsules
5. 2 tablets

Exercise 4

1. 4ml
2. 2.5ml
3. 4ml
4. 125mg
5. 75mg
6. 12.5ml
7. 15ml

Exercise 5

1. 847mg
2. 27.5mg
3. 265mg
4. 108mcg
5. 4g
6. 6.5g

Exercise 6

1. 12 tablets
2. 8 tablets
3. 4 tablets

Further reading

Ashelford, S, Raynsford, J and Taylor, V (2019) *Pathophysiology and Pharmacology in Nursing.* London: SAGE/Learning Matters.

Jones, BR (2013) *Pharmacology for Student and Pupil Nurses and Students in Associated Professions.* Amsterdam: Elsevier Science.

Prydderch, SB (2019) Preparing pre-registration nurses to be 'prescriber ready': Aspirational or an achievable reality? *Nurse Education Today, 78*: 1–4.

Useful websites

www.bnf.org/products/bnf-online/

British National Formulary: this is a useful website on information on all types of commonly used drugs and free to download as a smart device application.

www.medicines.org.uk/emc

e-medicines compendium: provides up-to-date, approved and regulated prescribing and patient information for licensed medicines.

www.npsa.nhs.uk/

National Patient Safety Agency website provides information on patient safety, including medication.

Chapter 9

Death, dying and cultural practices within palliative and end-of-life care

Jane Crussell and Robert Murphy

NMC standards of proficiency for registered nurses

Platform 3: Assessing needs and planning care

Registered nurses prioritise the needs of people when assessing and reviewing their mental, physical, cognitive, behavioural, social and spiritual needs. They use information obtained during assessments to identify the priorities and requirements for person-centred and evidence-based nursing interventions and support. They work in partnership with people to develop person-centred care plans that take into account their circumstances, characteristics and preferences.

At the point of registration, the registered nurse will be able to:

3.1   demonstrate and apply knowledge of human development from conception to death when undertaking full and accurate person-centred nursing assessments and developing appropriate care plans;

3.3   demonstrate and apply knowledge of all commonly encountered mental, physical, behavioural and cognitive health conditions, medication usage and treatments when undertaking full and accurate assessments of nursing care needs and when developing, prioritising and reviewing person-centred care plans;

3.4   understand and apply a person-centred approach to nursing care, demonstrating shared assessment, planning, decision making and goal setting when working with people, their families, communities and populations of all ages;

3.5   demonstrate the ability to accurately process all information gathered during the assessment process to identify needs for individualised nursing care and develop person-centred evidence-based plans for nursing interventions with agreed goals;

3.6   effectively assess a person's capacity to make decisions about their own care and to give or withhold consent;

3.7 understand and apply the principles and processes for making reasonable adjustments;

3.8 understand and apply the relevant laws about mental capacity for the country in which you are practising when making decisions in relation to people who do not have capacity;

3.14 identify and assess the needs of people and families for care at the end of life, including requirements for palliative care and decision making related to their treatment and care preferences;

3.15 demonstrate the ability to work in partnership with people, families and carers to continuously monitor, evaluate and reassess the effectiveness of all agreed nursing care plans and care, sharing decision making and readjusting agreed goals, documenting progress and decisions made;

3.16 demonstrate knowledge of when and how to refer people safely to other professionals or services for clinical intervention or support.

Platform 4: Providing and evaluating care

At the point of registration, the registered nurse will be able to:

4.1 demonstrate and apply an understanding of what is important to people and how to use this knowledge to ensure their needs for safety, dignity, privacy, comfort and sleep can be met, acting as a role model for others in providing evidence based person-centred care;

4.2 work in partnership with people to encourage shared decision making in order to support individuals, their families and carers to manage their own care when appropriate;

4.3 demonstrate the knowledge, communication and relationship management skills required to provide people, families and carers with accurate information that meets their needs before, during and after a range of interventions;

4.6 demonstrate the knowledge, skills and ability to act as a role model for others in providing evidence-based nursing care to meet people's needs related to nutrition, hydration and bladder and bowel health;

4.7 demonstrate the knowledge, skills and ability to act as a role model for others in providing evidence-based, person-centred nursing care to meet people's needs related to mobility, hygiene, oral care, wound care and skin integrity;

4.9 demonstrate the knowledge and skills required to prioritise what is important to people and their families when providing evidence-based person-centred nursing care at end of life including the care of people who are dying, families, the deceased and the bereaved;

4.10 demonstrate the knowledge and ability to respond proactively and promptly to signs of deterioration or distress in mental, physical, cognitive and behavioural health and use this knowledge to make sound clinical decisions;

4.13 demonstrate the knowledge, skills and confidence to provide first aid procedures and basic life support;

4.14 understand the principles of safe and effective administration and optimisation of medicines in accordance with local and national policies and demonstrate proficiency and accuracy when calculating dosages of prescribed medicines.

Chapter aims

After reading this chapter, you will be able to:

- identify the key professional values, skills and attitudes that are required to deliver palliative and end-of-life care in the twenty-first entury from the student nurse's perspective;
- describe holism in relation to assessment and identify how palliative care differs from other types of assessment in nursing care;
- review communication strategies and techniques to improve patient-centred palliative and end-of-life care;
- examine the concept of a 'good death' required in the last days of life and in bereavement care.

Introduction

Dame Cicely Saunders (1918–2005), nurse, physician, writer and founder of the hospice movement, wrote: *You matter because you are you, and you matter to the end of your life. We will do all we can not only to help you die peacefully, but also to live until you die.*

Palliative and end-of-life care nursing encompasses both the 'science of nursing' – that is, symptom management – and the 'art of nursing' – that is, communication. The nurse needs to understand how to engage with these concepts and elements in order to provide dignified and compassionate care within the changing care landscape. This chapter builds on earlier chapters – in particular, those on professional values and practice, communication and professional skills, and person-centred care. It aims to describe the professional values, skills and attitudes that are required of student nurses to deliver palliative care and end-of-life care in contemporary society. It begins with an approach to define palliative care in an ever-changing landscape of health and social care within healthcare. This chapter is designed to help you explore the concepts and issues of holism and assessment in any clinical or other setting in view of recent palliative and end-of-life strategies.

This chapter will help you consider death and dying from the patient-centred perspective to assist the student nurse or those new to the challenges faced when in a ward or community setting. In this chapter, you will learn how to assess an individual from person-centred and integrated perspectives. This will include the patient's journey from hospital to home, including the psychological, psychosocial, spiritual and practical perspective. The concept 'total pain' will be used as an example of symptom management, as not everyone at the end of life may present with pain. This concept can help you to address the wider needs of those who have been diagnosed with a life-limiting illness.

Communication is the key to good person-centred integrated palliative care. Communication strategies and techniques to improve professional and patient care are needed to facilitate transparent, integrated and therapeutic relationships to improve and ensure self-awareness and best outcomes specific to palliative care and those reaching the end of life.

In the United Kingdom there is a diverse and complex cultural and religious population. Therefore, knowledge, appreciation and integration of the multicultural and spiritual aspects of care are important in modern nursing. Multicultural and spiritual care will be examined and explored relating to student nurse education to help you enhance the care you will provide in palliative and end-of-life care.

Finally, in the light of recent guidance from NICE (2015b) and other national bodies, the last days of life will be explored and the specific role of the nurse will be examined. This will be accompanied by a reflection on bereavement and the possible support that can be offered to those who have experienced a personal death.

Case study: Ahmed – Part 1

You are a first-year student nurse on an oncology ward. In the morning handover, one of the patients you are assigned to is called Ahmed, and it was noted by the team that he is withdrawn. Ahmed is a 36-year-old carpenter who has a diagnosis of metastatic pancreatic cancer. As you were doing the morning clinical observations and taking his blood pressure, Ahmed becomes tearful and says, 'the pain is too much' and follows this with a further comment that 'I am so worried about my family'.

Ahmed is married to Jennifer, and they have three children between the ages of 6 and 10 years. Jennifer later reveals to you that Ahmed has not spoken to her about his disease progression or plans for the children.

This case study will develop throughout the chapter in order to demonstrate the importance that healthcare professionals develop appropriate values, skills and attitudes in holistic assessment, effective communication strategies, and guidance and support required over the palliative phase and into the end-of-life phase for a patient. The activities are designed to help you explore your personal and professional values in relation to death and dying. As you read each question, keep the scenario in the background of your mind, and think what the possible solutions might be to Ahmed's challenges.

Palliative care, holism and assessment

Care during the palliative stage of a disease and for end-of-life care is frequently complicated and can be dependent on a number of factors that range from the physical, psychological, ethical, nursing/medical, and social, spiritual, cultural and financial/practical matters. The range of symptoms, and how patients, families and professionals perceive the experiences can vary (Maher and Hemming, 2014). Table 9.1 highlights the possible symptoms and complexities associated with a life-limiting disease.

Common symptoms	Possible complexities
Pain	Spiritual distress
Nausea	Family/carer distress
Breathlessness	Professional and team anxiety
Depression	Social distress
Confusion	Psychological distress
Constipation	
Terminal restlessness	
Fatigue	
Dehydration	

Table 9.1 Possible symptoms and complexities associated with a life-limiting disease

It is important to understand that symptoms vary according to the patient's diagnosis and prognosis. The complexities can be compounded and vary depending on an individual's situation within the clinical or other setting. Some areas need to consider *holism* as an example, and address the biophysical, psychological, social, spiritual and cultural challenges. Holistic elements do not only lie within the central concerns of patients (and/family/carers), but are also relevant and a matter of concern to the team who are caring for them. The term 'holistic' within nursing is a broad attempt to accomplish the goal of holistic patient-centred palliative and end-of-life care.

Holism, or holistic, originates from the Greek word *holos* and refers to an individual as a whole person. In healthcare, it is associated with the term 'whole person care' and is the relationship between the biophysical, sociocultural, psychological and spiritual dimensions of the human condition (Maher and Hemming, 2014).

The history and ideals of holism have been concerned with the multidimensional aspects of being human with all its challenges. There have been strong associations with palliative care and holism since the inception and incorporation of palliative care as a speciality in nursing. Baldwin and Woodhouse (2011) explain that nurses need to provide excellence in palliative care by building a rapport and a relationship with the patient/family/carers. This can be achieved through engagement and building a trusting relationship that instils confidence. It is essential to understand and demonstrate empathy and deliver a caring attitude to an individual's care situation. In addition, the nurse who uses a holistic approach should not reduce the individual to a disease label, but actually use the 'whole person' perspective to embody and assess the needs from a plethora of differential grounds. Thus, holism and its integration into palliative care involves assessing the individual patient's needs using the practitioner's innate ability. This practice will ensure that the patient is not viewed as a physical entity, but that when an individual has symptoms and is suffering, there are factors beyond the physical interaction that require further investigation and assessment. Therefore, assessing an individual's palliative care needs requires reviewing all aspects of their biophysical, spiritual, psychological/cultural, social (and their integration in relation to a holistic or 'whole person' perspective). This will ensure that the best possible outcomes are achieved to alleviate the individual's suffering. For example, when exploring if a patient is in pain, the use of the 'total pain' concept can be used to address the broader aspects of pain from a multidimensional perspective.

Dame Cicely Saunders was not only a champion of holism in her pioneering work in palliative care, but she also introduced the concept of 'total pain' (Clark, 1999). Within this concept, we become aware of the holistic dimensions to symptom relief.

Total pain

When addressing the physical or unmet needs of a patient and the wider family/carers, the use of the 'total pain' concept may be a way into the more complex issues by reviewing one symptom like physical pain. Therefore, the nurse acknowledges that the individual patient is in physical pain in their initial assessment and by addressing it, may in turn introduce themselves into a deeper narrative. This may give the assessor the opportunity to explore how the physical pain is exacerbated by psychological, spiritual (or not), or other components that may be causing the patient distress. This in turn leads to the beginning of a holistic assessment of the needs of that individual, from a singular symptom.

Holistic needs assessment

NICE (2004) advocates that the principles of palliative care should incorporate holism, and indeed defines palliative care as 'active holistic care', while integrating the holism concept to help guide nurses and other healthcare professionals to understand and promote the use of holistic types of assessments from a nurse-practitioner perspective.

Through the above, we have begun to introduce and explore how holism may be used via the concept of 'total pain' and how this may be integrated into an assessment of the unmet needs of an individual. If we think of our case study with Ahmed, above, and the complex questions that may ensue, by way of addressing this from practical and practice perspectives, we will begin to see how holistic assessments are achieved.

The National End of Life Programme (2014) encourages nurses in health and social care to develop their skills in holistic assessment and to use the holistic tools available. Further reading related to assessment tools can be found at the end of the chapter. Assessment tools vary in nature and range from the general to the specific – that is, from assessing generalised pain to assessing one symptom of pain. If you use the appropriate assessment tools, the outcomes for patients are generally improved (Maher and Hemming, 2014). Figure 9.1 provides links to some of the assessment tools available for palliative care. It is worth noting that there is a limited amount of published research for validated tools for a comprehensive holistic needs assessment in palliative care and they all have some limitations (De Souza and Pettifer, 2013). Nevertheless, a number of tools are available to the practitioner when addressing the unmet needs of their patient group.

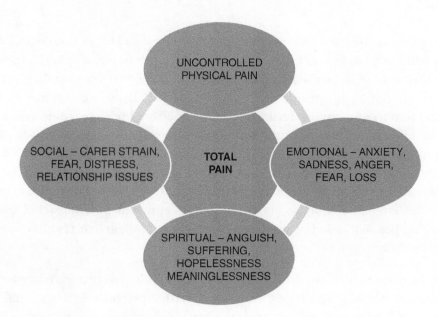

Figure 9.1 Total pain (Clark, 1999)

The Calgary–Cambridge model (Silverman et al., 2016) provides a structured framework to the initial consultation or meeting with the patient and may facilitate a relationship where the patient is made to feel comfortable and share information (Donnelly and Martin, 2016). It is worth noting at this point that a single assessment may not address all the unmet needs of a palliative care scenario, as this is dependent on the stage of the disease and prognosis. Therefore, the need to continually review and assess the patient's and the family/carer's unmet needs should be ongoing and continuous throughout the patient's hospital stay. The review and assessment process should be continued throughout the trajectory of the course of the disease and up to death.

Another tool that was designed within the Gold Standards Framework (Gold Standards Framework Centre, 2009) is the PEPSI COLA aide-memoire. This aide-memoire is useful for considering holistic domains and is a simple methodical way of assessing symptoms and can be used by the following acronym:

P – Physical

E – Emotional

P – Personal

S – Social Support

I – Information and communication

C – Control

O – Out of hours

L – Living with your illness

A – Aftercare

Each domain can be used as a prompt for the nurse to explore the needs of their patients and family in as much detail as required. For example, within the 'personal' domain the tool could be used to review what the individual's personal and cultural needs are in relation to spiritual/religious or specific dietary requirements. It may also help the nurse to explore further a patient's personal preferences in relationship to next of kin and decision-making around the individual's preferred place of care. Assessment tools such as PEPSI COLA do not need to be used in isolation and are not exhaustive in their assessment criteria in relation to palliative care holistic needs. The inclusion of other assessment aids can be incorporated – for instance, if the nurse is assessing the 'emotional' domain and it is noted that the patient is in psychological distress and has possible mood disturbances. An additional suggested resource would be the 'distress thermometer'.

A variety of assessment tools can be used to assess holistic palliative care needs. These tools measure physical symptoms, functional status, psycho–social–spiritual status and quality-of-life issues. Common tools used in palliative care can be accessed using weblink no. 2 to be found in Useful websites the end of the chapter. It is worth remembering that each tool should be assessed individually and evaluated for suitability to ensure a person-centred approach to care.

Psychological problems are common in palliative care patients. Fluctuations in feelings and mood, and living with uncertainty and doubt are the roads travelled emotionally when diagnosed with a life-limiting illness. For the novice nurse, when considering the assessment of a patient with psychological needs, it is worth bearing in mind the limitations of their role and signposting to other professionals within the multidisciplinary team. NICE (2004) recognises the different levels of professional psychological assessment and support. For first-year student nurses, the use of a recognised assessment tool is optional. These tools may help the nurse recognise the difference between a patient who is sad and one who is depressed. However, as indicated by the NMC (2015) *Code*, nurses should be aware of their limitations and refer the matter to an appropriate member of their team if the clinical assessment or complexity of the situation is outside their scope of practice.

When completing a holistic needs assessment, an important factor to take into consideration is the individual's mental stamina and their capacity to make informed decisions in relation to consent and treatment options. The mental well-being of the patient in palliative care can fluctuate and change suddenly due to a number of underlying pathophysiological reasons. Therefore, it is important that the nurse caring for a patient with a palliative progressive disease is aware of the Mental Capacity Act (2005). For further information, read *Law and Professional Issues in Nursing*, which is listed in Further reading at the end of the chapter.

The Mental Capacity Act (2005) was implemented in 2007 and governs how decisions are made for adult patients who lack capacity to make decisions for themselves. It also contains an assessment strategy or test for healthcare professionals such as nurses to fully comprehend when a patient lacks capacity.

It is worth noting that a person must be assumed to have capacity (to consent to or refuse treatments, or to make other care decisions), unless it is established that they lack capacity to make the decision in question. As mental capacity is decision-specific, when treatment options are offered – for example, as a disease progresses – the patient's mental capacity may need to be assessed each time a decision is introduced to the overall plan of care.

The responsibility for assessing and judging capacity lies with whichever professional is responsible for the decision-making process with the patient at the time. This could include, for example, a decision to feed a patient who is at risk of choking due to poor swallowing, or if their mental capacity deteriorates, and this has been discussed in previous meetings or consultation, or during Advance Care Planning (ACP). ACP will be discussed in more detail later in the chapter.

A single universal test can be used to ascertain if a person lacks capacity, if at the time the decision has to be made he has an impairment or disturbance of the mind or brain, and as a result they cannot:

- understand the relevant information;
- retain that information;
- use or consider it when making a decision;
- communicate their decision by any means.

These form the basis of the Mental Capacity Act (2005). Undertaking and being aware if someone has capacity to communicate effectively in decision-making is an important aspect in care delivery for a novice nurse. Communication and the challenges involved will be explored further in future sections of the chapter. However, before exploring the communications section, we will return to the case study above and explore some activities in relation to our discussion.

Considering the information you have been given about Ahmed, Activity 9.1 asks you to reflect on his situation and to explore some of the possible solutions to the questions. This activity aims to help you consider your own thoughts as you begin to experience caring for people at the end of their life.

Activity 9.1   Reflection

- How would you assess Ahmed's palliative needs using the concept of 'total pain'?
- Are there any specific tools of assessment that you may use?
- What are Ahmed's possible psychological needs and can you describe where he may be in relation to his family?
- How would you define his pain?
- How would you explore the possible solution for family or other support mechanisms for Ahmed?
- Does Ahmed have any spiritual or existential needs?

Some answers are provided at the end of the chapter.

Some of your answers to Activity 9.1 would involve communication with the patient, family and members of the healthcare teams. You will communicate differently with each of these groups, which will require different skills. In this chapter, we will focus upon communication directly related to palliative and end-of-life care.

Communication in palliative and end-of-life care

Everybody should have the opportunity for honest and well-informed conversations about dying, death and bereavement (National Palliative and End of Life Care Partnership, 2015).

Effective, honest, sensitive and compassionate communication is the cornerstone of good nursing care and a core element of *The Code* (NMC, 2015). It allows and encourages informed decision-making, focusing on priorities, wishes and hopes. When communication fails to be as effective as it could be, the outcomes can be misunderstandings, confusion, unmet needs, frustration and, potentially, harm.

Although highlighted in the press in 2015 that the UK provides the best palliative care in the world (Economist Intelligence Unit, 2015), a review in 2016 by the Care Quality Commission highlighted inequalities in access to palliative and end-of-life care and communication failures. Baroness Neuberger's review of the Liverpool Care Pathway in 2013, 'More care, less pathway', had previously made sweeping recommendation for improvement in end-of-life communications based on the public- and media-supported evidence of failings within the health sector to effectively and compassionately communicate with those requiring palliative and end-of-life care, and those important to them.

The Care Quality Commission (2016), NICE (2015), RCN (2015) and Age UK (2017) all highlight the essential need for effective communication through all stages of a person's journey in healthcare, but particularly when addressing needs within palliative and end-of-life care. There is agreement of the need for open, honest and compassionate communication, and an assumption that all people will benefit from early conversations. As the population is ageing and the age profile is growing larger, the Care Quality Commission (2016) suggest the focus for initiating conversations about a person's wishes and preferences for care as they near the end stages of their life should occur at an earlier phase rather than focusing primarily on the last 12 months of life, as often occurs. Earlier conversations and the ability to engage with ACP has been demonstrated to reduce costly and unhelpful care interventions, while improving patient and family-positive experience of care (Tavers and Taylor, 2016). ACP allows patients and those important to them to focus on their concerns, fears, hopes and wishes while they have capacity and reduces the decision-making burden on families and friends, as highlighted by Dehlin and Wittenberg (2015).

Despite understanding the pivotal role that communication plays in effective, compassionate and patient-centred palliative and end-of-life care, there are many reasons why communication can be problematic. Healthcare workers may feel they don't know what to say, develop a fear of upsetting people and families, or being blamed for the message being relayed. They may also fear the repercussions and a reaction for which they do not feel able to manage effectively. There may be feelings of failing the person or wanting to shield them. They may feel awkward about showing sympathy, feel powerless to control their own or the other person's emotional distress, and embarrassed about how to behave when someone is very upset.

A common reason for not wishing to engage in palliative and end-of-life conversations is lack of time within busy and challenging healthcare settings. These conversations can also highlight our own vulnerability and feelings around death and dying, which may be uncomfortable to explore. It is important, however, to take time to reflect upon your own feelings on death and dying, as understanding how your views will impact on any discussion is important. Any concerns and fears we may have can be transposed into our discussion and cause us to lead rather than support or advocate. Activity 9.2 below is designed to help you reflect on your views on death and dying.

Activity 9.2 Reflection

Take some time to reflect on your own feelings.

- What does death and dying mean to you?
- Have you ever discussed this before within your social sphere or family?
- Do you have fears, concerns?

Take some time with a colleague/supervisor/assessor to discuss your answers.

As the answers are based on your own observation, there is no outline answer at the end of the chapter.

Having taken time to reflect on your thoughts in Activity 9.2, we will now consider two main types of communication.

Verbal and non-verbal communication

Verbal communication includes rate of speech, quality, tone, pitch and volume of voice, the language used and types of questions. The way a question is phrased, timing and types are an important factor and some examples are provided below in Table 9.2. Taking time to formulate a questioning style may help to generate confidence in approach and elicit the answers needed within an assessment of care needs or an open discussion of ACP. Below are some examples of questioning styles you may find useful.

You can also use the elements developed more extensively and in more detail using the Transforming Nursing Practice 'Palliative and End of Life Care in Nursing'.

Question type	Example	Uses
Closed	'You are here to have a scan of your liver?' 'Did your family attend with you?'	This is used to confirm facts and provide a quick response. It often closes the conversation as it does not allow for expansion. It can be useful to find out if the patient is alone or not, and does not ask them to reveal too much about themselves.
Open	'Tell me about your pain.' 'How would you like us to help you?'	This allows the person to expand their answer and tell their story. It may be too open for some discussions as it may be too unfocused.

Leading	'Your family are aware that you are in hospital, aren't they?'	This type of question is often used to confirm information and is usually answered as a 'yes' or 'no'. Can lead the person and hinder a wider answer.
	'We have been discussing your pain management strategies – do you feel we have discussed your concerns adequately?	It can offer some structure to the question and allow the patient to narrow their focus.
Multiple	'Can you tell me about your concerns, how they affect you and how you wish the team to help you?'	If given in a list format, this question style can cause confusion and lead to incorrect answers and interpretation. To be avoided, particularly in conversations with persons with cognition and comprehension difficulties.
		If broken down more, these questions can be useful to assist patients and families to focus on elements they may not have considered in a systematic way.

Table 9.2   Examples of questioning styles

Non-verbal communication incorporates body language, head and hand movements, eye contact, posture, facial expression, touch and personal space, and can have different emphasis, depending on culture and nationality (Nicol and Nyatanga, 2017). Being self-aware may assist in creating a more confident approach and breaking down some of the communication barriers created through non-verbal means.

Listening

One of the key skills in communication is the skill of listening. Shipley (2010) identified that nurses who spent time with their patients listening to their story were perceived to be caring nurses. It is a skill sometimes taken for granted, but is an active process that requires you to pay attention and focus in order to be truly effective. By listening, you are able to assess and understand the patient's journey, and their understanding and processing of information. As you develop in your career, you will realise that being listened to makes patients and families feel valued and engaged. Active listening is a concentrated effort to listen, hear, understand and remember. It aims to improve communication and requires intense concentration to be effective. Often when we listen to someone speaking, we can be more concerned with how we will respond or reply, and often miss the messages and cues being sent by the speaker. Active listening requires the listener to focus on the verbal and non-verbal elements. It incorporates not just what is being said, but also how it is said, and the feelings being expressed verbally and non-verbally. This skill will help you to determine if the patient has distress within the physical, psychological, spiritual or emotional dimension, and address care and support appropriately (Dehlin and Wittenberg, 2015).

Activity 9.3   Reflection

Think about a time when you engaged in a communication where you felt the person was actively listening to you.

- How did you know they were actively listening?
- What did this feel like for you?
- What did the listener do to make you feel this way?
- Could you try this technique to see the impact?

As this answer is based on your own observation, there is no outline answer at the end of the chapter.

Having taken time to reflect on your active listening skills in this activity, we will now focus on the following areas which are so important in palliative and end-of-life care, such as hope and cultural components.

Hope

Hope is an essential element of psychological wellbeing if patients are to experience relief, quiescence and balance throughout the trajectory of their disease (Clayton et al., 2008).

As a student nurse, you will be exposed to death and dying situations where hope is of great comfort to patients and their families. Hope is an important element in communication in palliative and end-of-life care. Patients and their families have identified a need for hope from those providing care (Clayton et al., 2008). Although it may seem contradictory to discuss hope within this context, patients and those important to them need hope to provide an ability to cope and meet the difficulties they will face within an uncertain future and health journey (Hawthorn, 2015). In end-of-life care, hope can be related to aspects of care such as hope for effective symptom management, hope to see a loved one, or hope to be able to see a sunrise. Maintaining a focus on patients' goals and wishes will foster a sense of hope and help to maintain meaningful engagements between all parties (Hawthorn, 2015). It is important not to give false hope, such as hope for a cure, but honest, open and compassionate communication with all members of the family and team can support a hopeful and meaningful end-of-life experience (Hawthorn, 2015).

Barriers in communication

In your student nurse role, you will realise that there are many reasons that communication can be difficult concerning death and end-of-life care, and there will be barriers to overcome. Finding the right words, the right time or confidence to begin a difficult conversation about a person's wishes, expectations and aspirations *is* difficult. Don't be scared, as this can be a daunting prospect for anyone in healthcare, but particularly when starting your nursing as a student (RCN, 2015).

When patients, their families or healthcare professionals become anxious, barriers in communication may occur (Wittenburgh et al., 2016). Low levels of anxiety are a facet of everyday life and help us to focus, but heightened anxiety can lead to selectivity in what is heard and understood in communications (Dehlin and Wittenberg, 2015). The nurse needs to be aware and assess what information is being given, and how it is being received and understood. Good verbal and non-verbal communication using active listening and an appropriate questioning style with reflection on the discussion could be helpful.

Inclusivity and strategies for ensuring effective communication with communication barriers such as language, memory dysfunction, hearing loss and cognitive impairment must be identified. You can use a holistic approach to do this using an appropriate communication strategy which meets the needs of the individual.

Self-awareness is a skill needed to reflect upon non-verbal communication behaviours and avoid demonstrating any of the following:

- lack of eye contact;
- closed body language (crossed arms/legs);
- physical barriers (desks, folders);
- disinterest;
- not listening and avoidance.

Verbal behaviours discouraging engagement include:

- use of closed questions;
- leading questions;
- ignoring cues;
- normalising/minimising the impact of what is being said;
- giving information/advice or reassurance too soon;
- changing the subject.

Strategies to improve communication

I can make the last stage of my life as good as possible because everyone works together confidently, honestly and consistently to help me and the people who are important to me, including my carer(s) ('Every Moment Counts', National Voices, National Council for Palliative Care and NHS England, 2015).

It is imperative to engage with those in our care and those important to them, taking opportunities to engage in conversations as they arise rather than waiting for the 'perfect time'. This may never come, and time wasted may be lost forever. It is important to remember that end-of-life conversations can evolve over time. Decisions made can be altered and changed as conditions alter. Having honest, frank and compassionate relationships can facilitate on-going conversations to meet the personalised needs of all. Healthcare staff must ensure collaborative working practices with all members of the multidisciplinary team supporting patients and families to ensure that effective person-centred and partnership working practices with integrated care is achieved for all patients in a culturally sensitive and spiritually supportive environment.

The 'wish list' presented by London South Bank University pre-registration nursing students (Fallows et al., 2018) provides some prompts on how students and staff can begin end-of-life conversations and engage with Advance Care Planning.

Spirituality

Spirituality is a difficult concept to define and can be understood and interpreted by people in different ways or indeed denied by some as existing. In 2011, the Department of Health supported a systematic review of spiritual care at the end of life (DH, 2011) having identified a need to explore its meaning and provide guidance on supporting patients, families and staff. The chaplaincy service also produced their guidelines in 2015 (NHS Chaplaincy Guidelines, 2015) identifying *Best practice for providing excellent spiritual care*. The scope and meaning remains elusive in the literature, but concentrates on individual beliefs, values, traditions and practices, including relationships to self, family, others, community, society and nature (Milligan, 2011; Wittenberg et al., 2016). It can include religious beliefs and affiliations, but this is not always the case.

Spiritual care is a component of Dame Cicely Saunders's concept of 'total pain'. This needs to be sensitively assessed to avoid or anticipate possible causes of distress, anguish and hopelessness. She highlighted the spiritual domain and linked this to suffering and healing, with the WHO supporting this view. A diagnosis of a life-limiting illness can cause a variety of reactions from despair to personal growth and transformation. Some people will draw upon their own personal coping strategies or from within their families, communities, society or religions to gain meaning and progress. Others may feel despair, loss of a sense of meaning and purpose in life, and increased suffering (Milligan, 2011).

Nurses have a very important role to play in supporting patients, those important to them and colleagues to explore and assess spiritual needs, and this is something that must not be neglected. Effective communication is pivotal to this role and identified in the work of McSherry (2006) as using specific communications skills to facilitate. These are identified as:

- attentive/active listening: focusing on what is being said, picking up cues and being comfortable with silence;
- non-verbal communication: being self-aware and communicating compassion, honesty and sensitivity;
- presence or giving time: being with the person in the spiritual, physical and psychological sense.

These skills have been identified throughout this section and are areas that you can practise in order to enhance your ability to communicate sensitively, holistically and compassionately while using a person-centred approach.

Cultural components in palliative care, death and dying

Cultural sensitivity or cultural competence incorporates issues and concepts around spirituality, religions, ethnicity, gender and language (Dehlin and Wittenberg, 2015). Each person remains an individual within these concepts and no two people represent or duplicate each other identically. This means that it is important for nurses in all phases of practice to ensure that a holistic, individualised and person-centred approach is used. In palliative care we must identify death and dying first and then incorporate cultural influences (Nicol and Nyatanga, 2017). When you discuss death and dying in an open, honest and sensitive way, concerns, fears, wishes and hopes are likely to be discovered, and these may link into cultural practices or concerns. Further discussion would then highlight how best to support the person individually and within their cultural sphere. Not all people within a cultural group will follow set practices, so it is always best to ask the patient about their own cultural practices.

Case study: Ahmed

Three weeks from your first meeting with Ahmed and on a morning shift, you are again requested to look after him for the shift. On greeting Ahmed on your nursing round, you observe that he has lost a considerable amount of weight. He looks very thin (cachectic). As you begin speaking to each other, he tells you about his time as a child and is making inappropriate comments about what you are wearing.

Activity 9.4 below is designed to help you to explore and understand how a patient's mental state can change at the end of life and the impact of this on the family and the role of the nurse when communicating with all involved.

Activity 9.4   Critical thinking

- What are the possible physical symptoms/reasons for Ahmed's mental state?
- How would you assess his psychological well-being?
- What communication strategies might you use to engage with Ahmed and his family?
- Are there interdisciplinary team members who can support Ahmed and his family?

As this answer is based on your own observation, there is no outline answer at the end of the chapter.

This activity should help you to identify the physical, physiological, psychosocial and spiritual needs of the patient and their family members. It will help you to decide what support to provide in terms of maintaining therapeutic input and person-centred care. By doing this, you would be able to address both physical and emotional needs and preferences in a warm, caring and compassionate way.

A good death

Dame Cicely Saunders wrote: *How people die remains in the memory of those who live on.*

We have just one chance to get end-of-life care right and the way we, as health and social care staff, approach and support those going through this difficult process, is of paramount importance. By understanding our own perceptions of what constitutes a good death and reflecting with others will help us to prioritise how we communicate, assess and engage with our patients and their families on this last journey together.

In the reflective activity below, you will have the opportunity to consider your personal and professional perceptions around death and dying, and the actions you will take.

Activity 9.5   Reflection

Reflect with a colleague/supervisor or assessor what would constitute a good death for yourself, a member of your family or a patient in your care.

- Do you feel there are differences in the needs between these groups?
- Why do you think this?
- Will this influence your choices/actions and if so how?

As this answer is based on your own observation, there is no outline answer at the end of the chapter.

The Leadership Alliance for the Care of Dying People (2014) sets out five priorities for the care of dying persons (see Table 9.3) and provides a framework to support staff to meet the complex needs of those who are dying. It highlights recognition as the first priority, as this is an area that can be difficult to identify and is highlighted by Taylor et al. (2017). Recognising the dying phase is not an exact science and can be very difficult and emotional for all involved. If a person deteriorates, they must be sensitively and appropriately assessed by a suitably qualified clinician, and the outcome of the assessment communicated to the person (if conscious) and those significant to them to ensure that their best interests are served (Leadership Alliance for the Care of Dying People, 2014).

1	Recognise	The possibility that a person may die within the next few days or hours must be recognised and communicated clearly, decisions made and actions taken in accordance with the person's needs and wishes, and these are regularly reviewed and decisions revised accordingly.
2	Communication	Sensitive communication takes place between staff and the dying person, and those identified as important to them.
3	Involve	The dying person, and those identified as important to them, are involved in decisions about treatment and care to the extent that the dying person wants.
4	Support	The needs of families and others identified as important to the dying person are actively explored, respected and met as far as possible.
5	Plan	An individual plan of care, which includes food and drink, symptom control and psychological, social and spiritual support, is agreed, co-ordinated and delivered with compassion.

Table 9.3 Priorities for the care of the dying person: roles and responsibilities of health and care staff

I suspect that we all would wish for a 'good death', but the concept is difficult to define (Nyatanga, 2016). It is often culturally and socially influenced and personally defined, and individual preferences regarding death may shift during a person's life or illness. *End of Life Care Strategy* (DH, 2008) identifies that patients want to be treated as individuals with dignity and respect. They want to be free from pain and symptoms, and to have control, autonomy and independence within a familiar environment. They may also want to be surrounded by those important to them, as these are elements that comprise a good death. Taking time to communicate effectively with persons who have been diagnosed with a life-limiting illness and those supporting them at the earliest possible stages may help to facilitate this much sought-after goal.

The goals for the end phase of a person's life are defined as the patient's comfort, and being peaceful and dignified with positive memories. ACP is a useful way of exploring and documenting these goals and preferences for end-of-life care. It is a voluntary process and should include areas such as the person's individual concerns and wishes, and the values and goals they identify as most important for them. It is also important to elicit the person's understanding of their illness and prognosis, which will help when discussing their preferences and wishes for what type of treatment is available and beneficial for them in the future. ACP should be addressed as early as possible in the disease trajectory. Development of an ACP can occur at any time and within any discipline. It should be encouraged to facilitate the wishes and wants of the person and their families before deterioration or difficulties in articulation and decision-making occur. However, if this has not been explored at this stage, it might be good time to begin to explore the patient's preferences when you first meet them. Development of ACPs facilitates collaboration and open, transparent and truthful communication.

Recognising the last days of life

Recognising that a person is dying is the first and most important step to being able to plan and prepare all for the end stages of a life. It is often a complex assessment of the patient's condition as being irreversible and based on a multidisciplinary discussion and agreement. Cancer patients have a more predictable disease trajectory than others with chronic conditions such as chronic obstructive pulmonary disease (COPD) and dementia, and, with an increasingly elderly population, this complex and challenging group are the healthcare picture we are most likely to see. It is important for health-care staff to identify this phase to enable targeted support and information to the person and their families, with the emphasis shifting from cure to maximising comfort. Once the last days are identified, the plan of care can be tailored to the specific needs of the dying person and family.

Signs and symptoms of death approaching

- Profound weakness – bed-bound.
- Diminished intake of food and fluids.
- Drowsy and/or reduced cognition.
- Gaunt appearance.
- Difficulty swallowing.

Hui et al. (2014) categorised the approach of death into early and late signs: the early signs category is defined as occurring within the week before death.

Some of the signs in this category are: decreased level of consciousness and the inability to mobilise independently or at all, to exercise, to be self-caring or to maintain oral fluid and food intake. These early signs are related to and are dependent on disease progression.

The late signs category is defined as occurring within the last three days: diminished pulses on the radial artery. The pulse may be intermittent, faint or difficult to feel. Respiration may be laboured with obvious movement of the jaw or lip pursing. Decreased urine output, noisy or Cheyne-Stokes breathing. Breathing may also be intermittent with apnoeic periods and you may observe peripheral discoloration.

Dying is a unique event for each individual with the focus on maximising comfort. Based on the content and activities within this chapter, particularly around assessment and communication, you should be able to identify the person's preferences and wishes through using the identified resources.

Using the ACP, appropriate assessment and effective communication tools as highlighted earlier in this chapter can help you to recognise signs and symptoms of dying. This in turn will help you to dynamically plan individualised holistic care effectively.

Symptom management

The main focus when the last days of life have been identified are considerations of continuation or discontinuation of interventions and what are the benefit/burden risks to the patient. The aim must be to minimise the burden and maximise the benefit. New or worsening symptoms may occur in isolation or in clusters and require continuous regular assessment to manage them to ensure that comfort is maximised. The basic principles of symptom control are to identify and reverse, if possible, biological cause, identify and reverse, if possible, psychosocial/spiritual causes and, if indicated, use appropriate medications correctly. The patient must be reassessed continually to monitor effectiveness or need for alternative management strategies. Communication between members of the multidisciplinary team, the person and their important others can assist this.

The five most common symptoms in end of life are pain, nausea/vomiting, dyspnoea, anxiety/delirium and noisy respiratory secretions. Management is assisted by the use of subcutaneous medications to maximise benefit and minimise the burden. Other challenges include dysphagia, constipation, urinary incontinence/retention, dry mouth and poor skin integrity.

Care after death

Being able to provide care after death is a uniquely privileged experience, but can be quite a difficult one if you are engaging with this process for the first time. Previously called 'last offices', this has been renamed to reflect the multicultural society in which we live and to encompass not just tasks required after death, but focusing on care of the deceased and those important to them.

The difficult-to-face fact for us all is that we are all going to die, but the manner and circumstances of that death are different for everyone. Some deaths are expected following illness, while others are sudden and unexpected. Age, sex, gender, culture, race, ethnicity and political affiliations do not deter death, but those providing care after death need to incorporate all the elements that made the person who they were in life holistic and inclusive after death.

Hospice UK (2015) published the following guidelines for staff responsible for care after death:

- Respecting the religious or cultural wishes of the deceased and their family where possible, and ensuring that legal obligations are met.
- Ensuring timely verification of death.
- Preparing the deceased for viewing, where appropriate, and supporting the family.
- Offering family present the opportunity to participate in the process and supporting them to do so.

- Ensuring, where relevant, that families are informed about the need for a post-mortem examination and given information about tissue retention and disposal methods.
- Preparing the deceased for transfer to the mortuary or the funeral director's premises.
- Ensuring that the privacy, dignity and respect of the deceased are maintained at all times.
- Ensuring that the health and safety of everyone who comes into contact with the deceased are protected.
- Facilitating people's wishes for organ and tissue donation.
- Returning the deceased's personal possessions to their relatives.

Death can occur in a variety of different places such as hospitals, nursing homes, hospices, homes, homeless shelters, the streets, in mental health services and prisons, to name but a few. Irrespective of where or how death occurs, providing care after death is part of ensuring that a person has a 'good death' as outlined above. Compassionate and effective communication skills are required to support the family, friends, community and carers of the deceased. An array of professionals are involved in care after death, such as doctors, nurses, mortuary staff, porters, ambulance staff, police, pathologists, funeral directors, chaplains and faith leaders (Hospice UK, 2015). Effective and sensitive coordination between these services is required to allow the family to grieve and not to be caught in confusions and miscommunications or processes that may cause these. This is our one chance to get it right.

While it is very important to care for the deceased and their loved ones, it is important for the healthcare professional to care for themselves as well. Nursing carries a high emotional labour quotient (Delgado et al., 2017) and requires development of emotional resilience to avoid emotional and caring fatigue. Seeking support and supervision when providing care after death for the novice nurse is very important to help develop the necessary skills and carry out the best care possible.

Personal care after death is dependent on where the person dies and the circumstances surrounding their death. A resource for staff responsible for care after death is available from Hospice UK (2015), which provides guidance on care after death, coronial requirements and personal care after death. For the novice nurse, it is important to have a supportive mentor who can facilitate the development of care after-death skills as a positive and rewarding experience (Pesut and Greig, 2018). They go on to say that providing good care at this difficult time aids nurses' coping strategies on their grieving process and will help to create meaningful experiences following death. Sensitive support of the family is very important at this time, as it can be very distressing for those close to the deceased to be unable to provide culturally and religiously sensitive care until the coroner has provided agreement.

If there is no requirement for coronial enquiry, personal care can be provided in line with the person's wishes or those of the family/important others. Some family members will want to be involved in providing personal care and this should be facilitated if possible.

Providing personalised faith care is also an important component of good care after death. Supporting and valuing the wishes of the deceased and those important to them is complex and individualised. A useful resource is provided by Public Health England (2016) (see Useful websites, link no. 6).

For further information related to deaths requiring a coroner's investigation, see:

Ministry of Justice (2014) *The Guide to Coroner Services and Coroner Investigations* (see Useful websites, link no. 5).

Public Health England (2016) *Faith at End of Life: A Resource for Professionals, Providers and Commissioners Working in Communities* is a very useful resource to help provide the best information and care for people and families with death, dying and bereavement (see Useful websites, link no. 6).

Chapter summary

Holism is concerned with 'whole person care'. Holistic needs assessment involves the use of the qualitative innate qualities of the nurse, as well as the more quantitative measures by the use of tools to address the unmet needs of their patient group. The Mental Capacity Act (2005) is an important aspect in assessment, as the mental capacity of palliative patients with progressive illnesses can fluctuate.

Communication is the cornerstone of nursing and is especially important in supporting patients, those important to them and healthcare staff to have meaningful discussions fostering open, honest and compassionate relationships. There are barriers to be overcome, but use of successful strategies can help these to be effectively managed and support collaborative relationships and meaningful engagements. Inclusion of spiritual and cultural needs assessment and understanding will help to individualise the care provided and meet wishes, hopes and expectations, and lead to a good death for the patient and those important to them.

A good death is an individualised concept and is dependent on a variety of factors. It is important to recognise that death is approaching in order to ensure that support is provided to meet the changing needs of the patient and those supporting them. Carers' needs must be taken into consideration, as loss and grief can be difficult for all to manage. Good supervision and support from supervisors and assessors will help the novice nurse to engage with care of the dying and the bereaved. Guidance is available for support of faith practices and the practical aspects of providing care after death. Nurses are in a uniquely privileged position in the palliative and end-of- life care for their patients and families.

Activities: Brief outline answers

Activity 9.1   Reflection (p214)

Please note these are suggestions and the answers are not exhaustive in their outcomes.

To assess Ahmed's palliative needs, reflect on the 'total pain' concept via the diagram given in the text and place his physical pain in the centre. Now trace his psychological/issues. He is tearful and expressing worries about his family. Therefore, he appears in psychological pain/distress. There is also a social component to his pain as he is separated from his family and is not exploring his disease progression with them.

With further assessment, exploration and questioning, you can ascertain if there is a spiritual component to his pain. You now can see by using this concept that it is a doorway to assessing some of the complex challenges he may be experiencing.

To further explore and assess the possible unmet needs of Ahmed, review the tools discussed in the text. By now, you should be thinking in a holistic manner and how these assessment tools can help you in your assessment. Remember to be critical and think about the limitations of the tools, and how assessment needs to be continuous throughout Ahmed's disease trajectory and up until his death.

With regard to Ahmed's psychological needs, as a novice nurse you need to be aware of your limitations with regard to the NMC (2015) *Code* and in the light of NICE (2004) guidelines for psychological support for Ahmed and his family. You may have perceived and think that indeed Ahmed may have psychological pain. You now need to ask yourself how you can help. This is where escalation to a more senior professional or with a specialist may be required to meet Ahmed's needs. Reflecting and discussing openly with your supervisor or a senior nurse may suffice – for example, they may suggest a referral to a counsellor or psychologist with Ahmed's consent.

To explore the possible solution for Ahmed's family or other support mechanisms, consider why he has not spoken to his wife about his disease progression. Could he possibly be overwhelmed by his disease progression or are his physical symptoms stopping him from reflecting on the present? Have the senior team not explored or informed him about his disease progression? Is his coping mechanism denial? You need to reflect on these questions and think what you would do. Again, be aware of your limitations and who you think you should escalate this to – perhaps escalate Jennifer's worries to your supervisor or senior nurse. They may suggest exploring a family conference to ensure that all concerned are up to date with relevant information. A family conference usually involves team members from across the healthcare disciplines to ensure that as many unmet needs as possible are captured in one meeting.

Further reading

Howatson-Jones, L, Standing, M and Roberts, S (2015) *Patient Assessment and Care Planning in Nursing.* London: SAGE/Learning Matters.

This book introduces student nurses and novice practitioners to the assessment process enabling them to identify patient problems in order for solutions to be planned and implemented. The book encourages critical thinking and urges students to consider the social, cultural, psychological and environmental factors, as well as the physical symptoms that may be present when making assessments.

Nicol, J and Nyatanga, B (2017) *Palliative and End of Life Care in Nursing.* SAGE/Learning Matters.

This text covers areas handling bereavement, cultural and ethical issues, delivering care in a wide variety of settings, symptom management and also ensuring your own emotional resilience.

This book is specifically designed to equip nursing students and non-specialists with the essential knowledge in relation to the care and management of people nearing the end of life.

Walshe, CE, Preston, NJ and Johnston, B (2018) *Palliative Care Nursing: Principles and Evidence for Practice.*

Palliative Care Nursing is essential reading for nursing students, professional nurses and other health and social care professionals providing supportive and palliative care to those with advanced illness or who are towards the end of life. This third edition of the acclaimed textbook has been extensively revised and examines important research studies, key debates around care and strategies to advance palliative care nursing.

In four sections, the book covers key elements of nursing practice towards the end of life:

- Defining the palliative care patient.
- Providing palliative nursing care.
- Caring around the time of death.
- Challenging issues in palliative care nursing.

Useful websites

1. *Advance Care Planning: It All Adds Up.* Available from:

   www.endoflifecare.nhs.uk/search-resources/resources-search/publications/acpguide.aspx

2. Assessment tools which can be used to assess holistic palliative care needs:

   www.npcrc.org/content/25/Measurementand-Evaluation-Tools.aspx

3. Assessing Distress: Caresearch:

   www.caresearch.com.au/caresearch/tabid/2950/Default.aspx#dist

4. *Finding the Words*:

   www.endoflifecare.nhs.uk/search-resources/resources-search/publications/imported-publications/finding-the-words.aspx

5. Ministry of Justice (2014) *The Guide to Coroner Services and Coroner Investigations.* Available from:

   www.gov.uk/government/publications/guide-to-coroner-services-and-coroner-investigations-a-short-guide

6. Public Health England (2016) *Faith and the End of Life:*

   www.gov.uk/government/publications/faith-at-end-of-life-public-health-approach-resource-for-professionals

Chapter 10 Contemporary issues in nursing

Peter Jones

NMC Standards of Proficiency for Registered Nurses

This chapter will address the following platforms and proficiencies:

Platform 1: Being an accountable professional

Registered nurses act in the best interests of people, putting them first and providing nursing care that is person-centred, safe and compassionate. They act professionally at all times and use their knowledge and experience to make evidence-based decisions about care. They communicate effectively, are role models for others, and are accountable for their actions. Registered nurses continually reflect on their practice and keep abreast of new and emerging developments in nursing, health and care.

At the point of registration, the registered nurse will be able to:

1.14 provide and promote non-discriminatory, person-centred and sensitive care at all times, reflecting on people's values and beliefs, diverse backgrounds, cultural characteristics, language requirements, needs and preferences, taking account of any need for adjustments.

Platform 2: Promoting health and preventing ill health

Registered nurses play a key role in improving and maintaining the mental, physical and behavioural health and well-being of people, families, communities and populations. They support and enable people at all stages of life and in all care settings to make informed choices about how to manage health challenges in order to maximise their quality of life and improve health outcomes. They are actively involved in the prevention of and protection against disease and ill health and engage in public health, community development and global health agendas, and in the reduction of health inequalities.

At the point of registration, the registered nurse will be able to:

2.7 understand and explain the contribution of social influences, health literacy, individual circumstances, behaviours and lifestyle choices to mental, physical and behavioural health outcomes.

Platform 3: Assessing needs and planning care

Registered nurses prioritise the needs of people when assessing and reviewing their mental, physical, cognitive, behavioural, social and spiritual needs. They use information obtained during assessments to identify the priorities and requirements for person-centred and evidence-based nursing interventions and support. They work in partnership with people to develop person-centred care plans that consider their circumstances, characteristics and preferences.

At the point of registration, the registered nurse will be able to:

3.4 understand and apply a person-centred approach to nursing care, demonstrating shared assessment, planning, decision making and goal setting when working with people, their families, communities and populations of all ages.

Chapter aims

After reading this chapter, you will be able to:

- identify key demographic changes which are likely to affect the nature of nursing in the coming years;
- describe the challenges and opportunities caused by patterns of migration;
- discuss ways in which as we live longer, healthcare provision in the United Kingdom will change;
- describe the key features of dementia;
- discuss the challenges to society and nursing if dementia becomes an even more common condition, as is predicted;
- discuss the causes and management of delirium.

Introduction

Case study: Looking to the future

2039: The author of this chapter is now 80 years old. On waking up, I reach out for my exo-skeleton, a set of reinforced clothes that support my muscles and bones. I pull them around me and fasten them up and, with its help, stand up. I have a Community Manager, born in Somalia and now working for the NHS, without whom I would be stuck, but she has 20 other clients and won't be able to see me until later. I FaceTime

(Continued)

(Continued)

her to say I am OK. With my exo-skeleton, I walk to the kitchen. I wobble a little and the carpet will send a message to the local physiotherapy centre to come round to see me later. In the kitchen, there is a screen which, on my arrival, says good morning and tells me to take the tablets for my heart, my arthritis and my forgetfulness. I talk easily to this robot which can assess my mood (grumpy normally) and reacts accordingly.

After breakfast, I spend the morning chatting to a fluffy mechanical seal that gently squawks as I stroke it and I feel much less grumpy. When, later, I decide to go for a walk outside my flat, my little bracelet with a satellite navigation device sends a message to my daughter to warn her that I am out and about.

The future will never be quite what we expect, and life in 2039 might well be nothing like this. But all the devices that have been mentioned in the case study above are either available now or being developed, and might, for reasons we will discuss later, become a big part of our professional and personal futures.

This chapter opens with an exploration of some likely changes to the make-up of the United Kingdom's population over the next two decades, and it will explore how the consequences of these changes might impact on the nursing profession. We will then look at migration and the ways in which meeting the differing needs of increasingly diverse populations make nursing more challenging. Next, the concept of healthy ageing will be examined. Following this, there will be a discussion of the causes and management of dementia. Finally, we will explore some approaches to nursing people with a delirium.

Thinking about the future

If a modern nurse were to read the nursing textbook (Pearce, 1971) that I used as a student, they would almost certainly find much of it very familiar. There is a core of nursing practice that will only change if human physiology changes. However, there have been enormous developments in nurses' clinical lives in the last 40 years, many of which have been driven by technology. However, over the last 50 years, the society in which we practice has also changed, and this trend will inevitably continue, almost certainly in unexpected ways, affecting nursing profoundly as it progresses.

The most recent National Health Service policy guide (*Five Year Forward View*, NHS England, 2014) makes some assumptions about the immediate future. The plan assumes that long-term conditions, like dementia, diabetes and heart disease, have become the dominant causes of ill health, involving 70 per cent of healthcare provision (this might change if infections resistant to antibiotics become more common).

As patients, people with long-term conditions tend to want full involvement in making decisions about their care, and they want care that is more fully integrated and responsive to their changing needs. Instead of people having to adapt to the needs of the health service, the health service will have to adapt to the needs of its users. All this is likely to take place in an economic environment in which health is becoming increasingly expensive and resources more limited.

Taking an even longer view, the booklet *Time to Think Differently* (King's Fund, 2013) sets out to predict the key issues affecting the health of people in the UK in the decades ahead. The authors made a set of observations. First, the population is likely to grow over the next 20 years (2012–2032) by 8 million to just over 61 million people. This population will be much more diverse. It is predicted that by 2031, 15 per cent of the population in England and 37 per cent of the population in London will be made up of people from ethnicities different from the majority white population. The nature of these people's lives will be different, too. By 2032, the authors predict that 40 per cent of all households will be people living alone. In particular, the number of people over 85 living on their own is expected to grow from 573,000 to 1.4 million.

It is believed that by 2040, nearly one in seven people will be 75 or older. It is thought that the increasing proportion of older people in society will be off-set to some extent by migration, which brings younger people into the country. If this prediction is correct, then it is likely that because older people tend to use health and social care services more, these services will have more work to do – and there will be a smaller pool of younger people to provide the workforce. Older people tend to suffer from a collection of ailments, which is called multimorbidity. This usually means that their illnesses are interconnected, complex and require more skilful responses from clinicians.

The risk of developing dementia increases as we age, so it is probable that, unless real breakthroughs in prevention are made, in future there will be more people with dementia to care for. No doubt nursing will rise to this challenge and others that are not yet known about. It will be an interesting journey.

Migration

The UK, already a diverse society, particularly in our cities, has recently received, and will probably continue to receive, increasingly large numbers of migrants from many different countries. Jayaweera (2014) suggests that from 1991 until mid-2014, migration contributed to just over half of the total population growth. Nurses are expected to understand and address the needs of these people. Many nurses, some perhaps reading this book, will come from these very same groups of migrants and, eventually, in their turn, will come to play leading roles in the health services.

Abubakar et al. (2016) have suggested that migration has become one of the key worldwide health issues, causing problems but also creating opportunities. It is emphatically not a recent phenomenon (the UK as a nation has a long history of immigration: Huguenots in the seventeenth century, Jewish refugees from Eastern Europe at the turn of the last century, workers from the Caribbean after the Second World War). But it is a phenomenon that appears to be accelerating, linked to both European Union rules around freedom of movement and to recent wars that have forced huge numbers of civilians from their homes. This movement of people into Europe in general does give the chance, if the problem is approached with compassion and imagination, to improve the health of these migrants. But migration also affects the host population by putting demands on existing health services, pressures which will no doubt be felt by future generations of nurses. And this might continue well into the future. Abubakar has written that *migration can have intergenerational effects. Migrants tend to adopt the health profile of their host population, but differences in health can persist for generations through biological, social, cultural, and economic determinants* (p141).

Rechel and colleagues (2013) and Zarb et al. (2012) warn that it is difficult to make robust generalisations about the health of migrants because the term includes such a wide range of people and experiences. They do, however, identify some apparent trends. Rechel et al. (2013) say that migrants when they first arrive in their new country are often healthier than the indigenous population – the 'healthy migrant' effect. This is usually because only fit and active people can manage the tough journeys involved. However, this good health does not always last.

Migrants seem to be more vulnerable to certain health problems. Western-style diets can be devastating for people brought up without fast-food outlets and ready-made meals. Some studies – for example, Zarb et al., 2012 – suggest that it is the children who suffer most, often leading to high levels of obesity. Studies have shown too that groups of people who have moved to Europe have higher levels of fat in their diet. Patel et al. (2006) found that Gujurati migrants to Britain ate foods with a higher fat and sugar content than their equivalents who remained in India. Because of this, type 2 diabetes can be a particular problem for migrant groups. Certain communicable diseases are also more common within migrant groups. Tuberculosis is an obvious example. Its spread is almost certainly linked to the crowded living conditions in which many of the less well-off migrants are forced to live. Migrant mothers too seem to do worse than women from the host population, with reports of higher levels of perinatal problems.

Because migrants tend to work long hours in low-paid and often more dangerous jobs, they tend to have worse occupational health experiences than indigenous populations. They also continue to work when they are unwell, worsening their condition and health.

Zarb et al. (2012) tentatively suggest that migration is a risk factor for schizophrenia. The migration process can be, as many news reports have graphically described, a very traumatic one and can lead to ongoing psychological consequences. Women and children seem to be at particular risk of traumatic events, possibly involving the experience of being trafficked for sexual exploitation. This can have a damaging effect on mental health (Jayaweera, 2014).

Because migrants can have very different genetic heritages, different groups seem to be more or less susceptible to different non-communicable diseases (non-infectious illnesses). For example, migrants from Africa and the Caribbean are more likely to die from their stroke than Europeans. They are more prone to hypertension and diabetes, but not to coronary heart disease (Zarb et al., 2012).

There is some evidence that migrants have problems negotiating their way around unfamiliar health systems. Jayaweera (2014) identifies several reasons for this. First, insufficient information about healthcare systems in the UK can make getting to health services particularly difficult for newly arrived migrants. Almost inevitably there will be language barriers and there are often problems accessing translators. Migrants, struggling to get an economic toe-hold in the country, can find the cost of transport to hospital appointments prohibitive. Many live in areas of deprivation where services may be thin on the ground. It has been reported that migrants are often unaware of their rights to access the National Health Service. And, sadly, on occasions, incidences of cultural insensitivity by staff have occurred.

Issues around migration will be significant ones for the next generation of nurses to manage. As Jayaweera (2014) has identified, care can be compromised by cultural insensitivity or lack of knowledge by clinicians. It is important that nurses are not barriers to good quality care, but actively reach out to migrants. The diversity of the nursing workforce should facilitate this. But cultural sensitivity and a sound knowledge of the health issues facing migrants should be fundamental to twenty-first-century nursing.

Some issues arising from an ageing population

The fact that people are living longer is a sign that we are leading healthier lives and this trend is likely to continue, although it is not inevitable. In the UK, the increase in life expectancy is slowing down more quickly than in other similar countries (Public Health England, 2017). However, good health in later life is not shared out equally. Inequalities in health across the lifespan continue and this means that poorer people are not benefiting in the same way as their wealthier neighbours.

Concept summary

Our understanding of what 'old' is has changed over time. Elaine Cumming and William Henry in their book *Growing Old* (1961) suggested that old age is characterised by older people voluntarily withdrawing from an active involvement in society (disengagement theory). This view was contested in Robert Havighurst's alternative

(Continued)

(Continued)

understanding of successful ageing (Havighurst, 1963). He found that older people want to remain involved in society, and it is society that does not allow them to do this. If they could remain active citizens, they would have healthier and more fulfilled lives. Robert Atchley (1989) suggested that it was wrong to mark old age as a great divide in people's lives. He found older people wanted to continue with those interests they enjoyed earlier in their lives. In 1997, Rowe and Kahn identified the factors that lead to successful ageing. This influenced the World Health Organization's Active Ageing initiative (2002) with its 'three pillars' of participation, health and security.

While generally the health of older people is improving, this is not true for everyone. Old age can be a time of increasing ill health. A King's Fund report (2013) states that the number of people with some specific age-related diseases will double over the next 20 years. For example, by 2030 there will be 17 million people with arthritis and 3 million with cancer. The report also states that the number of people suffering from co-morbidities – that is, more than one long-term condition – will grow rapidly. And worse, increasing numbers of people will have three or more long-term conditions. This increasing presence of co-morbidity in the ageing population will inevitably take a toll on how well these people can manage in their daily lives. Consequently, by 2030 the number of older people with care needs is predicted to rise by 61 per cent (King's Fund, 2013).

Scenario: Polypharmacy

Because older people frequently have co-morbidities – a number of long-term problems – they often need very complex drug regimes. Taking four or more medications is called 'polypharmacy'. This is often unavoidable because the patient needs each drug, but they can often cause problems for older people. Taking so many drugs can be unpleasant and difficult. There can also be unwanted interactions between the different chemical compounds as the drugs are broken down in the body. Drumbeck et al. (2015) investigated this issue. They looked at three common conditions: heart failure, type 2 diabetes and depression. The authors then imagined these patients suffering from nine other common illnesses on top of these. Following accepted clinical guidelines, the authors identified the drugs that were recommended to treat each of these conditions. If these drugs were used for people with type 2 diabetes, the authors identified 133 potentially serious drug interactions that could arise when treating the nine co-morbidities. For patients with depression, 89 possible adverse reactions were identified. This article shows clearly the potential hazards in treating some very common conditions with commonly used drugs.

It is not simply that we give older people too many drugs. There is evidence, too, that older people are also not given medicines that would help them. There is a guideline called Stopp/Start used in the NHS which aids effective prescribing for older people. As more nurses now have a prescribing role (O'Mahony et al., 2015), they take on the responsibility to ensure that their prescriptions for older people really are beneficial.

It is perhaps helpful to break down old age into two rather different parts. First, from the age of retirement to the age of 75 (it is very hard to be precise) is seen as a relatively benign time of reasonable health, reasonable wealth and a pronounced social engagement. This has been called the 'third age'. People in this group go on cruises to the Caribbean, help as volunteers in local hospitals, and care for their grandchildren and less well older friends and relatives.

Potentially, the greatest challenge facing those involved in looking after older people will be to try to prolong this third age of good health and well-being for as long as possible. The term 'compression of morbidity' (Fries, 2002) has been used to describe this. Patterns of illness suggest that people tend to have a period of worsening health in the two years or so before they die. The hope is that we can really squeeze this period of ill health right back into people's lives and keep them fit and healthy for as long as possible. There is evidence to suggest that in the UK we can get much better at this. In order to achieve this compression of morbidity, we need effective public health measures to keep us as healthy as possible throughout our lives, not just when we reach old age. Bernard Isaacs (1924–1995) coined the phrase 'the geriatric giants': instability, immobility, incontinence, intellectual impairment/memory and impaired independence (Isaacs, 2002). These certainly have not gone away and compressing morbidity still largely means keeping these at bay.

Case study: My father's co-morbidities

When I think about my father's life, I can see this effect. He had been a very active man throughout his life, but a series of events happened to him in the last three years before he died. He began to have transient ischaemic attacks because of an underlying atherosclerotic disease. We felt he was unsafe at his home and he moved to live with my family. He then began to have a series of urinary tract infections, probably linked to a mildly enlarged prostate. He lost the sight in one eye to glaucoma. He then began to fall, probably rushing to a toilet when not being able to see clearly. And we began to get to know the local paramedics and become regular visitors to our nearby hospital's Accident and Emergency Department. Finally, he suffered a stroke from which he did not recover, but he stayed with us throughout. Despite this being quite a tough time, it was also a particularly enjoyable one with much more laughter than sorrow.

A new approach to our health issues has developed in the past decade, which is the idea of frailty management. Fried et al. (2001) have suggested that frailty is a *biologic syndrome of decreased reserve and resistance to stressors, resulting from cumulative declines across multiple physiologic systems, and causing vulnerability to adverse events* – that is, our bodies work less well as we age and a relatively minor infection or fall can tip us over the edge into a much more serious illness. One of the key features of this is sarcopenia, a decrease in muscle bulk and strength. Frailty is, alongside dementia, long-term conditions and multimorbidity, one of the key concepts in how we look at the care of older people. In essence, it means that we intervene energetically at any sign of a decrease in an older person's ability to care for themselves in order to keep them as independent as possible.

The care of older people takes place in a variety of interconnected environments: primary care, with GPs and district nurses, secondary care in acute hospitals and supported living in rest and nursing homes. To make matters more complicated, a new range of services, sometimes called intermediate care, have evolved. These involve organisations that aim to prevent an admission to a hospital bed, or to allow a patient to be discharged home as quickly as possible. Clinicians often need to think very carefully about what is the best choice for their older patients.

There is plenty of evidence to suggest that an acute hospital admission may not always be the right place for older people (Keeble et al., 2019). They can lose strength and the ability to care for themselves during a hospital stay, as well as being at risk of falling, catching an infection or becoming delirious (more of this later). So, it is vital that older people are only admitted into hospital when we know that it will benefit them, and that they should stay there no longer than is strictly necessary.

The World Health Organization's Active Ageing programme (WHO, 2002) is perhaps the best-known global approach to developing healthier lives for older people. The underpinning principles of human rights, equity, equality and non-discrimination (particularly on the basis of age), gender equality and intergenerational solidarity are very important alongside the central strategy of promoting the active involvement of older people in society. Activity 10.1 now asks you to reflect on meeting the needs of older people.

Activity 10.1   Reflection

The World Health Organization has a list of eight domains that need to be addressed in order to meet the needs of older people. What do you think these are?

There is an outline answer at the end of the chapter.

As we saw in Activity 10.1, older people's good health is influenced by broader social issues, as the WHO Active Ageing approach makes clear. Health in old age is also enormously dependent upon how well you have been across the course of your earlier life. Even so, in a variety of settings, good nursing care in a patient's later years will have profound and positive effects on their on-going health and well-being.

Dementia: an approach to care

The next part of this chapter will be a survey of dementia. This is partly because it is important for us all to understand dementia. Also, and perhaps of more importance in the context of this chapter, it is because dementia can act as an exemplar for modern nursing practice.

Burns and Iliffe (2009) define dementia as *a clinical syndrome characterised by a cluster of symptoms and signs manifested by difficulties in memory, disturbances in language, psychological and psychiatric changes, and impairments in activities of daily living.* Kitwood (1997) suggests that the way the syndrome progresses depends on a cluster of factors: personality, life experiences, concurrent health and well-being, and the environment of the person with dementia. These profoundly alter the course of the central disease, which damages the person's brain. Dementia is now the most common cause of death in the UK for women and the proportion of those dying from dementia is increasing (Office of National Statistics, 2017). When someone is older than 65, the risk of developing the most common kind of dementia, Alzheimer's disease (AD), is 1 in 14. If you live to be 80, this rises to 1 in 6. One million people in the UK will have dementia by 2025, and this will probably increase to 2 million by 2050 (Alzheimer's Research UK, 2017).

The skills needed to manage dementia are similar to those in managing all long-term conditions, which is a feature of modern healthcare. There are several reasons for this. Dementia is a chronic illness that involves management across primary, secondary and social care. It is a condition that features several transitions. On one hand, it involves moving around different clinical environments. On the other, the person experiences profound changes in their range of actions and abilities as the syndrome progresses. The nursing role is often facilitative, helping the patient and their loved ones to achieve the goals *they* want to achieve. It involves a good understanding of the relevant clinical evidence and good communication skills so that nurses can help clients make good decisions. Often the patient and their carers are the experts in each individual case, and the nurse needs both a level of humility to acknowledge this and the ability to know when more directive support is needed. Teamwork around the patient will involve many members of the interdisciplinary team, and this interdisciplinary working is increasingly a model for medical care provision.

Preventing dementia

Medical science has not yet discovered the cause of Alzheimer's disease and because of this, we have not developed curative drugs. Instead, there is now a developing emphasis on dementia prevention by good public health. This approach was laid down in the Blackfriars Consensus of 2014, which placed dementia within the family of non-communicable diseases and suggested that broad health prevention measures and good brain health across a person's lifespan are an effective way to address the 'dementia crisis'. Activity 10.2 asks you to think about how you can give health promotion advice

Activity 10.2   Critical thinking

A friend of yours is about to have a child and she asks you about how she can try to limit the risk of her child developing dementia in later life. She wants to know what she can do herself and what advice can she give her child when they are growing up. This is possibly a slightly strange question, but how would you reply?

An outline answer is provided at the end of the chapter.

After completing Activity 10.2, you will have identified the risk factors for dementia. According to Wise (2017), if a specific set of risk factors are adequately addressed, 35 per cent of dementias can be prevented. The risk factors are familiar: hypertension, obesity, smoking, physical inactivity and diabetes, which all seem to increase the chance of developing dementia. In addition to these, a history of depression, a lack of education in early life, deafness, sleep disorders and social isolation have also been identified as specific risk factors. It is known too that continuing involvement in education, exercise, social interaction in religious or other groups and a good diet can reduce the risk or limit the severity of dementia.

Although the WHO's Active Ageing initiative is not essentially about dementia, the underpinning principles of human rights, equity, equality and non-discrimination (particularly on the basis of age), gender equality and intergenerational solidarity have a particular resonance in addressing dementia-centred issues. Addressing gender issues is a particular priority. Corfield (2017) has pointed out that dementia is a particular issue for women, both because more women suffer from dementia than men globally (lack of educational opportunities and the chance to build up the all-important cognitive reserve in global terms might be a major issue here) and also because women tend to be the main caregivers, both informal and formal.

In the UK there are two sets of dementia-specific government-led strategies. The dementia strategy *Living Well with Dementia* (DH, 2009) was the first, setting a range of ambitious outcomes, but essentially with three overarching goals. These are to improve public and professional awareness of dementia, to diagnose the problem early and quickly start supportive interventions, and finally, to help people live well with dementia.

A second initiative, the *Prime Minister's Challenge on Dementia* (2015) followed hot on the heels of the dementia strategy. The challenge set outs two sets of goals for the UK.

First, *for the country to be the best country in the world for dementia care and support and for people with dementia, their carers and families to live,* and second, to be the best place in the world to *undertake research into dementia and other neurodegenerative diseases.* Activity 10.3 asks you to consider the barriers to engaging in community roles for people with dementia.

Activity 10.3   Reflection and critical thinking

What barriers do you think prevent people with dementia from taking a bigger role in their community? List three potential barriers.

An outline answer is provided at the end of the chapter.

Dementia subtypes

From completing Activity 10.3, you should have a better understanding of the barriers to community engagement for people living with dementia. NICE (2018) recommend that when someone is diagnosed with a dementia, they should be told their subtype. There are many different kinds of dementia. Robinson et al. (2015) list the most common: Alzheimer's disease (50 per cent of cases), vascular dementia (25 per cent), frontotemporal dementias, dementia with Lewy bodies (15 per cent) and Parkinson's disease with dementia. It is possible to identify some common symptoms. The most widely recognised is memory loss, but there are many others. People with dementia can have difficulty concentrating, they may find it hard to carry out familiar daily tasks, such as getting confused over the correct change when shopping. They may struggle to follow a conversation or find the right word, and can become disorientated. People with dementia can become prone to rapid mood changes.

There are, however, significant differences between the various types of dementia. For example, people who live with Lewy body dementia may often experience hallucinations, in the same way as those suffering from Parkinson's disease, and the two conditions share many features (Guerreiro et al., 2016). Frontal lobe dementia can lead to more marked personality and language changes (Warren et al., 2013). But it is more important to know the person with dementia and not to nurse a diagnosis.

Diagnosis and management: NICE guidelines

The National Institute for Health and Care Excellence has recently published a set of guidelines on how to manage dementia (NICE, 2018). First, underpinning everything else, they recommend a collaborative approach to care not only involving people living with dementia in decisions about their care, but also an approach where a clinician actively seeks feedback from the patient and their family to ensure that they are providing care appropriately. One of the moral imperatives here is to get informed consent for any action carried out with the patient. Informing the patient in ways that are appropriate to the patient's level of understanding will certainly put demands on nurses' inventiveness and creativity.

While a national screening programme for dementia is not recommended (Robinson et al., 2015), it is probably true that early diagnosis, one of the key outcomes in the dementia strategy, is beneficial to people with dementia and their families. Memory clinics have become the place where diagnoses of dementia are formally made (Kelly, 2008). The clinics try to make a rapid diagnosis, having ruled out the presence of other, potentially treatable, medical conditions such as a brain tumour or hypothyroidism.

Objective cognitive assessments tools are key to the process. NICE (2017) recommend a selection of tools that have a strong evidence base. Probably the most common tool used is the Mini Mental State Examination (MMSE). This 30-question screening tool asks the client to undertake a range of small cognitive tasks and produces a score that identifies the presence, and degree, of any cognitive problem. It is not diagnostic in itself and requires the person administering the test to be aware of other factors that might give a false idea of the patient's capabilities – for instance, English might not be the person's first language or they might have hearing or motor problems.

If a positive diagnosis is made, a care plan should be developed for the person with dementia, and if necessary a care package of support started. After diagnosis, people with dementia and carers *are often baffled by the complexities of the health and social care systems* (Design Council, 2014). NICE suggest that the newly diagnosed person with dementia should have one named care coordinator to help them navigate their way through such a complicated set of services. It is recommended that patients should be told of their rights to have an advocate at any consultation to support them. Their care plan, too, should be one that follows the patient around so that an accurate record is available to newly involved clinicians.

Patients may be offered the opportunity to go to support groups providing cognitive stimulation or reminiscence therapy. Occupational therapy might be needed in order to help the patient function effectively in their activities of daily living (ADLs).

Later, as the syndrome worsens, people with dementia can experience a common set of problems. Dementias finally affect all aspects of the person's life. Memory problems tend to worsen so that people may not recognise close family and friends. NICE (2018) recommend reminiscence therapy and group cognitive stimulation to help maintain cognition (thinking ability). Communication problems can become pronounced. Some people may eventually lose the ability to speak altogether. People with dementia may begin to have considerable difficulties moving around and struggle to remain continent. Both appetite and weight loss problems are common. Many people have trouble eating and swallowing food and fluids, which can lead to choking, drooling and chest infections (Burns and

Iliffe, 2009). All these problems should be addressed as energetically as the person with dementia wishes. Close working with dieticians and good bowel management are important. Smaller, softer, more frequent meals may be appropriate. The input of a speech and language therapist, occupational therapist and physiotherapist may all be beneficial throughout the progression of the dementia (NICE have published a set of guidelines on managing the symptoms of dementia (2018), depression (2018) and incontinence in women only (2015), whose principles can serve as the bedrock of our care).

Behavioural and psychological symptoms of dementia (BPSD, or behaviours that challenge) tend to worsen as the dementia progresses. These may include increased agitation, depressive symptoms, anxiety, wandering, aggression or sometimes hallucinations. These issues can often lead to family or informal carers feeling that they cannot continue to look after a patient in their home. In the UK, Admiral Nurses who work in the community, support both the person with dementia and their loved ones in managing these problems, or help the family group to develop coping strategies. One approach is to look for possible causes of the behaviour – for instance, pain, thirst, hunger, infection or boredom – and then try to address the issue. Carers can look for trigger points that may provoke certain actions and try to avoid these. Door alarms can be fitted to prevent patients from wandering outside or themselves be fitted with tracking devices, although these can cause some ethical problems. Each individual case will need its own solutions.

These behaviours are challenging for trained clinicians to manage effectively when working in a team with breaks and easily available support. Isolated family or informal carers with 24-hour responsibilities deserve professional understanding and support to help them through these extremely demanding experiences.

Since Dr Alois Alzheimer first labelled the disease in 1907, three clinical features of Alzheimer's disease (AD) have been identified. First, the formation of amyloid *plaques* disrupting neurotransmission. The formation of these plaques is controlled, to some extent, by certain genes. A second feature of AD are Tau-protein *tangles* around the brain cells which are thought to damage the axons. Third, in AD, there are significant changes in the effectiveness of neurotransmitters. In particular, the acetylcholine cholinergic pathways are compromised. This observation has led to the creation of a family of drugs that slow the breakdown of acetylcholine in the brain (acetylcholinesterase, AChE inhibitors). There are three formulations of these drugs, *donepezil, rivastigmine* and *galantamine,* in common use. Acetylcholinesterase inhibitors can modify the progress of the disease, but they are not a cure and have a limited *window of effectiveness* (Rodda and Carter, 2012). This means that, for reasons we do not quite understand, they work for a certain length of time and then sadly begin to become less effective.

Another feature of the role of neurotransmitters in AD is excitotoxicity, an overexposure to another neurotransmitter called glutamate, leading to the loss of damaged neurones. *Memantine,* the second drug type used in AD, works by blocking glutamate receptors within the brain (Briggs et al., 2016). This can be used alone or alongside the AChE inhibitors.

Drug regimens are different if the person with dementia does not have AD. Donepezil, Rivastigmine or Memantine can be used for those with Lewy body dementia, but not in vascular dementia, unless an element of AD is present. Prescribers should be very careful to avoid the use of anticholinergic medication whenever possible. These drugs appear to worsen dementia symptoms. NICE suggests that antipsychotic medication can be used for patients who are very distressed or hallucinating, but only when other management methods have been tried and failed. In general, the advice is not to use medication for problems like sleeplessness or depression, but to use non-pharmacological approaches. Pain is a more common feature of dementia than is commonly thought. Normally, a self-reporting pain assessment tool is the best approach to use, but in severe dementia an observation pain assessment tool, like the Abbey pain chart, can be used, observing behaviours, facial expressions and movement as clues to the person's level of discomfort. Pain management then should proceed with caution, but using the normal range of analgesics.

People with dementia in hospital

NICE highlights the problems that arise when a person with dementia is admitted into hospital. These transitions in the lives of people with dementia can be problematic, and the care of people with dementia in acute hospitals has become an area of intense practice development. People with dementia tend to stay in hospital longer and have more accidents. Patients are not only being admitted because of a primary diagnosis of dementia, but more commonly because of a concurrent health problem – for example, falls, diabetes, strokes, urinary tract infections or chest infections.

The Alzheimer's Society, in a survey of acute hospital care in 2016, reported that their respondents found there was a frequent lack of respect shown towards the person with dementia when they were admitted to hospital. Hospitals were widely perceived as being frightening places. A huge majority of the respondents (90 per cent) said the person they knew with dementia became more confused while in hospital. So, this transition, from home to hospital, needs to be managed extremely carefully. The Royal College of Psychiatrists (RCPsych, 2017) recommends a range of interventions to achieve this. First, nurses should look out for, and promote the use of documents like the Alzheimer's Society's leaflet 'This is me'. This is completed by the carers of a person with dementia, documenting their life story and individual preferences and habits so that, even when the patient cannot talk about themselves, nurses know enough about them to provide care which recognises the patient's individuality. The RCPsych audit (2017) identified mealtimes as being particularly problematic. This suggests that flexible support was needed for meeting the eating and drinking requirements of people with dementia because they might not want to eat at more conventional or regular times, or at a socially accepted speed.

The audit also found that people with dementia were still not being included as fully as possible in making decisions about their care. This was despite the powers of the Mental Capacity Act (2005) which had created a framework within which people with cognitive and communication difficulties are empowered to make decisions. Clearly, hospitals need to find ways to create an environment in which people with dementia are allowed to make choices and have a level of autonomy. NICE (2018) recommends that the Mental Capacity Act should be a staff training priority.

Recently, a pressure group has started John's Campaign which promotes co-caring of people with dementia while they are in hospital, so that the presence and involvement of family members enables the person with dementia to see familiar and comforting faces.

Many hospitals now set out to be dementia friendly with careful use of colour coding to identify toilets, eating areas and sleeping parts of the ward. The University of Stirling has an interactive site which suggests how hospitals can be designed with the patient with dementia in mind.

A tool that can be used in working with people with dementia is validation therapy (VT). This has perhaps rather taken over from reality orientation (RA) as the key clinical and therapeutic approach to care. RA tried to pull people living with dementia into the world as experienced by clinicians and carers by reminding the person with dementia constantly what the time was, where they were geographically and correcting 'errors' in the person's thinking. Validation therapy, on the other hand, asks carers to enter the world of the person with dementia on their own terms. The aim is to create a, perhaps fleeting, moment of empathetic communication and warmth. At its heart is an attempt to find out what is meaningful in the life of the person with dementia and engage with this. There is a well-known example of this on the internet, showing the woman who developed the idea, Naomi Feil, demonstrating it perfectly (see the link in the Useful websites section at the end of the chapter). An example of how validation therapy can inform common nursing actions is explored in the following activity.

Activity 10.4   Reflection and critical thinking

A common experience when working with people with dementia is finding a way to help an anxious patient who is searching for a family member or feeling that they should be somewhere else, and that other people will be missing them.

You might in practice be approached by a person who is well into their nineties telling you that they need to get home because their mother is expecting them home for tea. They are clearly desperately anxious about this.

1.   If we were following the therapeutic approach suggested by reality orientation, how would we deal with this behaviour?

2.   If your approach was based on the idea of validation therapy, how would you approach differ?

An outline answer is provided at the end of the chapter.

Activity 10.4 would have helped you to understand therapeutic approach and valida-tion therapy. The most important element of a successful hospital stay, however, will be the approach taken by the nurses and other clinical staff. Perhaps the key thinking in the development of dementia-sensitive nursing practice was by Tom Kitwood who developed two key ideas. First was the notion of 'malignant social psychology'. This is where the actions of carers harm the health and well-being of the person with demen-tia. Kitwood's concern is that carers should not do anything to worsen the condition of the person with dementia. This obviously excludes any unprofessional or abuse activ-ity, but also Kitwood warns about being overly protective, taking away choice, treating the person with a dementia as you would a young child (Kitwood, 1997). Kitwood also writes about positive things: allowing the person with dementia the opportunity to be active, to express their emotions, to feel part of the ward community and, most impor-tantly, to remain an individual. All this should be alongside the warm, positive regard, compassion and patience shown by the nursing team.

Inevitably, dementia care will, finally, involve end-of-life care, and this is another focus of nursing practice development. In their survey of the literature on end-of-life care for people with dementia, Lillyman and Bruce (2016) have identified a number of crucial issues. First, a clear recognition is needed when the person with dementia enters the last stage of their life. This is important both for the person with dementia and perhaps even more so for the family and loved-ones. The Alzheimer's Society suggests that the following symptoms are useful markers to help identify when a person with dementia is reaching the end of their life. The patient may be deteriorating more quickly than before, they may lose consciousness, become unable to swallow, agitated or restless. An irregular breathing pattern may develop (this can be dramatic like Cheyne-Stokes breathing – increasingly deep breaths followed by long pauses) and there may be a more marked cooling of hands and feet. This seems simple, but this stage may be the culmination of an extended, very gradual process and it can be easily missed.

When people with dementia reach the end of their lives, ethical problems and dilem-mas may come to the fore. It is much easier to provide good end-of-life care to people if you know what their wishes were for their last days rather than having to second-guess them. If this has been achieved, then some of the complex ethical issues will become much less fraught. The National End of Life Care programme (2014) has published a clear guide of ways in which this can be achieved. First, people can write an Advanced Care Plan which *tells other people, friends and family, the GP about their wishes*. This is not legally all-powerful, but it gives clinicians a sense of what the person wants. Second, the person with dementia can write an advanced decision to refuse specific treatments in specific circumstances. This requires some skill and legal formality. It must be wit-nessed and is legally very compelling. It does not, however, allow a patient to specify what care they do want. *A Lasting Power of Attorney* order formally appoints someone to speak or act for the person with dementia once they have lost the ability to make or communicate their own decisions. There are two sorts of attorney. One gives per-mission to an attorney to manage financial issues. The other allows the attorney to make healthcare decisions on behalf of the patient with dementia. When the person with dementia is dying, the attorney would be central in deciding the appropriate care for that person. It is an enormously responsible role (National End of Life Care programme, 2014*).*

The provision of comfort, managing symptoms effectively, reducing levels of pain, whether the cause is physical, spiritual, social or psychological, are central to good palliative care. This can become particularly problematic and demanding when the patient has a dementia and again calls on a specific skill set, which nurses working in this field will develop.

Delirium

Oh et al. (2017) state that delirium

> *is defined as an acute disorder of attention and cognition. It is a common, serious, and often fatal condition among older patients. Although often under-recognized, delirium has serious adverse effects on the individual's function and quality of life, as well as broad societal effects with substantial health care costs.*

Delirium is brought on by a possible trigger: an infection (chest infections and urinary tract infections are common causes), constipation, pain, dehydration, sensory over- or understimulation (there are many). Certain drugs can cause a patient to become delirious.

Delirium is characterised by a disturbance in attention and awareness. It has a rapid onset – either a matter of hours or days – and it can vary hour by hour. Cognition (the way the person thinks) changes and often the patient perceives his or her environment differently, frequently with some suspicion. A delirium is caused by a specific underlying medical condition or, on occasions, by a change in environment (Todd and Teale, 2017).

Case study: Mr Mullins

Mr Mullins is an 82-year-old man who has worked all his life in the building trade. He normally lives alone at home with minimal help from his family. He came into hospital for surgery on his cervical spine following a history of back pain. The operation went well, but his recovery was problematic. One day after surgery, he woke early and got out of bed, pulling his drip-stand with him. He accused the ward staff of trying to poison him and refused medication. He went back to his bed and fell into a very deep sleep, becoming quite hard to wake. A strong man, he raised his fists at anyone who came near him. At lunchtime, he appeared calmer and ate his food without a problem, but refused any medication. By the evening he was once again clearly distressed, walking around the ward and, on one occasion, threatening a nurse with violence.

(Continued)

(Continued)

At 10 o'clock at night, Mr Mullins was persuaded to take a sedative tablet. He slept well and in the morning was willing to take his normal medication including analgesia and antibiotics. Staff helped him to drink plenty of fluids. His family came in to sit with him. His behaviour became calmer and three days post-operatively, he was back his normal cognitive function.

This case study demonstrates many of the key characteristics of delirium – a rapid onset: changes in the patient's condition throughout the day, sometimes alert, sometimes showing an altered level of consciousness. Its cause may never be clearly known – unfamiliar surroundings, the anaesthetic agent, pain, dehydration – all could be responsible. In this case, the patient responds without any specific intervention. This does not always happen.

There are two kinds of delirium. First, hyperactive delirium, where the patient's actions are clearly different from normal, often involving combative behaviour and suspicion of staff members. Second, hypoactive delirium where the patient's behaviour is not obviously different although their thoughts may be muddled. This kind of delirium often gets missed because the patient is quiet, often drowsy, but usually cooperative with clinical staff. However, beneath the surface, their thoughts can be chaotic. Patients can veer between both kinds of delirium (mixed delirium).

Nurses, alongside clinical colleagues, have four goals in their work with delirium. First, they need to identify those at risk. Delirium can be a phenomenon in intensive care units and end-of-life care settings, but it is essentially associated with older people. Todd and Teale (2017) identify a set of risk factors. They find that one-third of patients over 80 years old in a general hospital will experience an episode of delirium, but suggest that even those as young as over 60 years are more at risk. This risk is increased if they have a problem with their hearing or eyesight, need help with washing or dressing, and possibly already have a diagnosis of dementia. Men are more at risk than women. If the patient is taking several different kinds of medication or is having orthopaedic surgery, their risk of developing a delirium is also increased.

After identifying those at risk, a second priority for nurses is to start an action plan. Inouye et al. (1999) have developed an approach to delirium management which is aimed at reducing the chance of an at-risk patient developing delirium in the first place. The evidence suggests that effective interventions should be tailored to the differing circumstances of each individual, but they are likely to include a pattern of actions. These involve orientating the patient to reality (this seems to work better in delirium than in dementia), achieving the right level of stimulation (lighting and noise levels are important here), encouraging mobility, facilitating good sleep patterns and encouraging the presence of familiar faces. It is hoped that by identifying those at risk and planning preventative measures, a case of delirium can be prevented. However, this is not always possible and, if a case of delirium does develop, it needs to be identified as quickly as possible. Delirium has been called a medical emergency because its consequences can be so severe.

A third priority for nurses is that once a delirium has been identified, the underlying cause should be treated as quickly as possible. The delirium will not go away unless this is achieved. NICE (2010) has developed a set of practice guidelines to inform clinical responses to delirium. These may involve managing pain, identifying the source of an infection and treating it with antibiotics, rehydrating the patient or correcting electrolyte imbalances. Whatever the cause, it must be treated aggressively.

Finally, nurses need to care for the patient with delirium in such a way as to minimise the person's distress by creating the best possible environment of care. This would again follow Inoye's environmental recommendations, as well as good nursing care and the minimal use of sedation or restriction of freedoms. Sometimes these are necessary if the patient puts their own health, or that of others, at risk (NICE, 2010). Nurses also need to support the patient's loved ones through what can be an extremely traumatic experience. Later, if they experience distressing flashbacks and memories, the sufferer will need support, too. These disturbing memories can linger far longer than is often appreciated by clinical staff.

Unfortunately, the consequences of suffering from a delirium can be profound, even when it is identified and treated quickly. Gross et al. (2012) identified that dementia patients who developed delirium were less likely to be alive two years later than their peers who did not. Salluh et al. (2015) found the same effect too when looking at the post-delirium health of very ill, non-dementia patients.

So, nurses have key roles to play all around: identifying those people who might be at risk of developing delirium then planning and implementing care in such a way as to reduce the risk of delirium. They need to rapidly identify patients who do develop delirium and treat them with compassion and skill, while playing their part in identifying the cause. This involves good communication with the patient, family and friends, and being realistic and informative about the possible lingering effects of the delirium.

Chapter summary

This chapter will have demonstrated, barring unexpected developments (good, or bad), certain ways in which nursing is likely to develop in the next few years. It has suggested that nurses in the twenty-first century will be faced by issues arising from increases in human longevity and changing patterns of migration. Nurses will need to develop skills in nursing an increasingly diverse community. They will be engaged in promoting good health across the lifespan and helping older people remain as active as possible throughout their later years. Readers will be aware of the NICE guidelines on managing dementia and their role in providing effective care to those affected by this, increasingly common, syndrome. A four-part approach to preventing recognising and treating delirium is also discussed, following NICE guidelines.

Activities: brief outline answers

Activity 10.1   Reflection (p238)

1. Outdoor spaces and building. These include access and safety, green spaces, walkable streets, outdoor seating and accessible buildings (lifts, stairs with railings).

2. Transportation, including accessible and affordable public transport, is a key issue for people in later life.

3. Housing and support that allows people in later life to age comfortably and safely within the community to which they belong are universally valued.

4. Social participation. It is important to enable people to exercise their competence, enjoy respect and esteem, and maintain or establish supportive and caring relationships. Enabling accessibility, particularly for those with mobility issues, is also key.

5. Respect and social inclusion. On one hand, many feel they are often respected, recognised and included, while on the other, they experience lack of consideration in the community, in services and in the family.

6. Civic participation and employment. Those options can include paid employment or voluntary work, if they so choose, and to be engaged in the political process.

7. Communication and information. Staying connected with events and people, and getting timely, practical information to manage life and meet personal needs is vital for active ageing.

8. Community support and health services. GP practices that work for older people help in balance training and keeping active and community services that work for older people.

(www.ageing-better.org.uk/age-friendly-communities/
eight-domains, accessed August 2018)

These domains are a gateway to understanding holistically the needs of older people. Healthcare is only a small part of this.

Activity 10.2   Critical thinking (p240)

1. Have a boy – women have a higher risk of developing dementia.

2. Do not pass down to your child in the genes you give them a particular variant of the gene apolipoprotein E (APOE) which increases a person's risk of developing Alzheimer's disease.

3. Tell your child to eat sensibly, especially fruit, vegetables and a little oily fish.

4. Tell your child never to take up to smoking, to get plenty of exercise throughout their life, to go to university and to keep studying throughout their life. Possibly tell them they have to learn to play the piano when they reach 70 in order to keep their brain active.

5. Tell your child to stay happy. Depression in later life is a risk factor for dementia.

6. Tell them to look after their eyesight and hearing; sensory loss can be a risk factor.

7. Tell them to be a joiner-in; being involved in a church or other social group reduces the risk of dementia, and tell them not to sit at home and mope. Social isolation is possibly a risk factor.

8. Tell your child not to drink alcohol or at least very little. This is an area of debate. On the whole, it is thought that alcohol is bad for the brain.

9. Do not drop your baby repeatedly on its head or suggest that boxing is a good career option; head injuries are a risk factor for dementia.

(Alzheimer's UK, 2016)

Clearly, this mother-to-be will not be able to influence many of these factors. She cannot choose to have only boys even if she wanted to, and certainly cannot control which genes she passes down. But good childhood health leading to a healthy lifestyle in an adult are clearly beneficial in maintaining good health generally, as well as in reducing the risk of developing dementia.

Activity 10.3   Reflection and critical thinking (p241)

Answers according to Alzheimer's UK survey (2013):

- a lack of confidence (69%);
- being worried about becoming confused (68%);
- being worried about getting lost (60%);
- mobility and physical health issues (both 59%);
- not wanting to be a burden to others (44%);
- lack of transport (33%).

These are the real worries of people with dementia preventing them from taking a more active part in community life. But as more people in every community will have dementia, communities are beginning to address the needs of people with dementia living in the community. See Useful websites below for the link to view an interesting BBC film on Bruges, which is seen as one of the world's leading dementia-friendly cities. It shows how the community is trying to deal with the anxiety, fear of being judged, or getting lost and confused that people with dementia may experience.

Activity 10.4   Reflection and critical thinking (p245)

In reality orientation, a nurse may be dragged into repeating the fact that the patient's mother must have died some years previously and could not possibly be waiting to give the patient their tea. This can not only cause distress to the patient, but my experience is that it is very unlikely to stop the patient worrying. Naomi Feil's approach would be to judge that this behaviour is demonstrating how strong is the patient's memory of her mother. Therefore, the approach might be: 'Tell me more about your mother. Was she very strict?' In this way, you can open an interaction that has real meaning for the patient, may cause pleasure in her recollections and break, even for a moment, the patient's sense of isolation.

Further reading

Gawande, A (2014*) Being Mortal: Medicine and What Matters in the End*. New York: Metropolitan Books/Henry Holt & Co.

A wonderfully readable, intelligent and thought-provoking book about how we care for older people; it is particularly thoughtful on end-of-life care. If you read one book on ageing, this is the one.

Koser, K (2016) *International Migration: A Very Short Introduction*. Oxford: Oxford University Press.

A concise account, suitable for the busy student.

Pachana, N (2016) *Ageing: A Very Short Introduction*. Oxford: Oxford University Press.

As the name suggests, this is a good short book on all issues of ageing.

Useful websites

These five websites have been chosen from among many. All of them will open doors to an overwhelming number of exciting and interesting developments in this chapter's topics.

www.ageuk.org.uk

Age UK: the leading British charity supports older people and their carers.

www.alzheimers.org.uk

Alzheimer's Society: a key charity that is all things to do with Alzheimer's disease.

www.bbc.co.uk/news/av/health-21516365/pioneering-dementia-friendly-community-in-bruges

BBC film of Bruges as a dementia-friendly city.

www.migrationwatchuk.org

Migration Watch, based at Oxford University, is a site that publishes well-researched briefing documents on aspects of migration.

http://dementia.stir.ac.uk

Stirling University Dementia Services Development Centre: a very attractive site with strong visual information, particularly on developing dementia-friendly environments.

https://youtu.be/VwIEbjJZKOg

Validation therapy: a powerful short film by Naomi Feil and Gladys Wilson of the potential of validation therapy.

http://apps.who.int/iris/bitstream/10665/67215/1/WHO_NMH_NPH_02.8.pdf

World Health Organization's Active Ageing initiative: a worldwide development promoting active ageing, age-friendly communities. A very strong European site too.

References

Abbey, J, Piller, N, Bellis, AD, Esterman, A, Parker, D, Giles, L and Lowcay, B (2004) The Abbey pain scale: a 1-minute numerical indicator for people with end-stage dementia. *International Journal of Palliative Nursing*, *10* (1): 6–13.

Abubakar, I, Devakumar, D, Madise, N, Sammond, P, Groce N, Zimmerman, C, Aldridge, R, Clark, J and Horton, R (2016) UCL–Lancet Commission on Migration and Health. *The Lancet*, *388*: 1141–2, 17 September.

Ackley BJ and Ladwig, GB (2014) *Nursing Diagnosis Handbook: An Evidence-based Guide to Planning Care* (10th edn). St Louis, MO: Mosby/Elsevier.

Adam, S and Osborne, S (2005) *Critical Care Nursing: Science and Practice* (2nd edn). Oxford: Oxford University Press.

Age UK (2017) *Let's Talk about Death and Dying – How to Have Difficult Conversations.* Available online at: www.ageuk.org.uk/globalassets/age-uk/documents/booklets/talking_about_death_booklet_final_version.pdf

Akın, A, Alp, E, Altındis, M, Azak, E, Batırel, A, Çağ, Y, Durmuş, G, Kurt, EK, Sağıroğlu, P, Türe, Z and Ulu, AC (2018) Current diagnosis and treatment approach to sepsis. *Mediterranean Journal of Infection Microbes and Antimicrobials*, *7.*

Allen, D (2009) The legacy of Project 2000. *Nursing Standard*, *23* (34).

Alzheimer's Australia (2014) *The Valuing People Framework.* Available online at: https://valuingpeople.org.au/the-framework/the-valuing-people-framework (accessed 12 April 2018).

Alzheimer's Research UK (2017) *Dementia Statistics Hub.* Available online at: www.dementiastatistics.org/ (accessed December 2017).

Alzheimer's Society (2016) *Fix Dementia Care.* Available online at: www.alzheimers.org.uk/download/downloads/id/2907/fix_dementia_care_-_hospitals.pdf

Alzheimer's Society (2017) *End of Life Care: Factsheet.* Available online at: www.alzheimers.org.uk/download/downloads/id/2907/fix_dementia_care_-_hospitals.pdf (accessed 20 November 2017).

Alzheimer's Society (2017) *Dementia Friends.* Available online at: www.dementiafriends.org.uk/

Andrews, JA (2014) *Trusted to Care: An Independent Review of the Princess of Wales Hospital and Neath Port Talbot Hospital at Abertawe Bro Morgannwg University Health Board.* Available online at: https://gov.wales/docs/dhss/publications/140512trustedtocare en.pdf (accessed 8 April 2018).

Atchley, RC (1989) A continuity theory of normal aging. *The Gerontologist, 29* (2): 183–90.

Badriyah, T, Briggs, JS, Meredith, P, Jarvis, SW, Schmidt, PE, Featherstone, PI, Prytherch, DR and Smith, GB (2014) Decision-tree early warning score (DTEWS) validates the design of the National Early Warning Score (NEWS). *Resuscitation, 85* (3): 418–3.

Baldwin, MA and Woodhouse, J (eds) (2011) *Key Concepts in Palliative Care.* London: SAGE.

Barrett, D, Wilson, B and Woollands, A (2012) *Care Planning.* Harlow: Pearson Education.

Bell, E, Campbell, S and Goldberg LR (2015) Nursing identity and patient-centredness in scholarly health services research: a computational text analysis of PubMed abstracts 1986–2013. *BMC Health Services Research, 15* (1). Available online at: https://doi.org/10.1186/s12913-014-0660-8.

Boore, J, Cook, N and Shepherd, A (2016) *Essentials of Anatomy and Physiology for Nursing Practice.* London: SAGE.

Breeding, M (2014) Web-scale discovery services. *American Libraries, 45* (1/2): 25–25, January/February.

Briggs, R, Kennelly, SP and O'Neill, D (2016) Drug treatments in Alzheimer's disease. *Clinical Medicine, 16*(3): 247–53.

Britten, N, Moore, L, Lydahl, D, Naldemirci, O, Elam, M and Wolf, A (2017) Elaboration of the Gothenburg model of person-centred care. *Health Expectations, 20* (3): 407–18.

Brooke, J, Cronin, C, Stiell, M and Ojo, O (2017) The intersection of culture in the provision of dementia care: a systematic review. *Journal of Clinical Nursing,* 9 August 2019. Epub.

Burns, A and Iliffe, S (2009) Clinical review: dementia. *BMJ, 338.* Available online at: www.bmj.com/content/338/bmj.b75

Businessballs (2017) *Brainstorming for Team Building and Problem Solving.* Available online at: www.businessballs.com/problem-solving-and-decision-making/brainstorming-for-team-building-and-problem-solving-how-to-109/ (accessed 14 February).

Care Quality Commission (CQC) (2016) *A Different Ending: Addressing Inequalities in End of Life Care.* Available from: www.cqc.org.uk/sites/default/files/20160505%20CQC_EOLC_OVERVIEW_FINAL_3.pdf

Carpenito-Moyet, L (2007) *Understanding the Nursing Process.* Philadelphia, PA: Lippincott Williams & Wilkins.

Castro, EM, Van Regenmortel, T, Vanhaecht, K, Sermeus, W and Van Hecke, A (2016) Patient empowerment, patient participation and patient-centeredness in hospital care: a concept analysis based on a literature review. *Patient Education and Counseling, 99* (12): 1923–39.

Cathala, X and Moorley, C (2019) Accountability as a newly qualified nurse. *Nursing Times* (in press).

Centre for Disease Control (2017) *Get Ahead of Sepsis.* Available online at: www.cdc.gov/sepsis/basic/index.html (accessed 20 February 2018).

Chabeli, MM (2007) Facilitating critical thinking within the nursing process framework: a literature review. *Health SA Gesondheid, 12* (4): 69–89.

Chapman, H (2017) Nursing theories 1: person-centred care. *Nursing Times, 113* (10): 59.

Clark, D (1999) 'Total pain', disciplinary power and the body in the work of Cicely Saunders, 1958–1967. *Social Science and Medicine, 49:* 727–36.

Clayton, JM, Hancock, K, Parker, S, Butow, PN, Walder, S, Carrick, S, Currow, D, Ghersi, D, Glare, P, Hagerty, R and Olver, IN (2008) Sustaining hope when communicating with terminally ill patients and their families: a systematic review. *Psycho-Oncology: Journal of the Psychological, Social and Behavioral Dimensions of Cancer, 17* (7): 641–59.

Clissett, P, Porock, D, Harwood, RH and Gladman, JR (2013) The challenges of achieving person-centred care in acute hospitals: a qualitative study of people with dementia and their families. *International Journal of Nursing Studies, 50:* 1495–503.

Coombs, T, Curtis, J and Crookes, P (2011) What is a comprehensive mental health nursing assessment? A review of the literature. *International Journal of Mental Health Nursing, 20:* 364–70.

Corcoran, N (2011) *Working on Health Communication.* London: SAGE.

Corcoran, N (ed.) (2013) *Communicating Health: Strategies for Health Promotion* (2nd edn). London: SAGE.

Corfield, S (2017) *Women and Dementia: A Global Challenge.* Available online at: www.ageinternational.org.uk/Documents/women_dementia_global_challenge_report.pdf

Cottrell, S (1999) *The Study Skills Handbook.* Basingstoke: Macmillan.

Crème, P and Lea, MR (1997) *Writing at University: A Guide for Students.* Maidenhead: McGraw-Hill/Open University Press.

Crook, H, Evans, J, Pritchard, B, Yates, A and Young, T (2014) *The All Wales Best Practice Statement on the Prevention and Management of Moisture Lesions.* The All Wales Tissue Viability Nurse Forum. London: Wounds UK.

Cumming, E and Henry, WE (1961) *Growing Old.* New York: Basic Books.

De Souza, J and Pettifer, A (2013) *End-of Life-Care.* London: SAGE.

Dehlin, O and Wittenberg, E (2015) Communication in palliative care – An essential competency for nurses. In Ferrell, BR, Coyle, N and Paice, JA (eds) *Oxford Textbook of Palliative Nursing* (4th edn). Oxford: Oxford University Press.

Delgado, C, Upton, D, Ranse, K, Furness, T and Foster, K (2017) Nurses' resilience and the emotional labour of nursing work: an integrative review of empirical literature. *International Journal of Nursing Studies, 70:* 71–88.

Department of Health (DH) (1997) *The New NHS: Modern and Dependable.* London: The Stationery Office.

Department of Health (DH) 1999 *Making a Difference: Strengthening the Nursing, Midwifery and Health Visiting Contribution to Health and Healthcare (Nursing Strategy).* London: The Stationery Office.

Department of Health (DH) (1998) *A First Class Service: Quality in the New NHS.* London: The Stationery Office.

Department of Health (DH) (2005) Mental Capacity Act. London: HMSO.

Department of Health (DH) (2006) *Modernising Nursing Careers: Setting the Direction.* London: The Stationery Office.

Department of Health (DH) (2008) *End of Life Care Strategy: Promoting High Quality Care for All Adults at the End of Life.* London: The Stationery Office.

Department of Health (DH) (2009) *Living Well with Dementia: A National Dementia Strategy.* London: The Stationery Office.

Department of Health (DH) (2011) Health and Social Care Bill 2011. Available online at: http://webarchive.nationalarchives.gov.uk/20130107105354/http://www.dh.gov.uk/en/Publicationsandstatistics/Legislation/Actsandbills/HealthandSocialCareBill2011/index.htm (accessed 4 April 2018).

Department of Health (DH) (2012) *Equity and Excellence: Liberating the NHS.* London: The Stationery Office.

Department of Health (DH) (2015) *NHS Constitution.* London: The Stationery Office.

Department of Health and Social Care (2016) *The Report of the Short Life Working Group on Reducing Medication-related Harm.* London: Department of Health and Social Care.

Design Council (2014) *Living Well with Dementia: A Design Council Challenge.* Available online at: www.designcouncil.org.uk/sites/default/files/asset/document/Living%20Well%20with%20Dementia%20Design%20Challenge%20Research%20Report.pdf (accessed 1 December 2017).

Donnelly, M and Martin, D (2016) History taking and physical assessment in holistic palliative care. *British Journal of Nursing,* 25 (22): 1250–5.

Dumbreck, S. Flynn, A, Nairn, M, Wilson, M, Treweek, S and Mercer, SW (2015) Systematic examination of drug-disease and drug-drug interactions following recommendations in 12 UK national clinical guidelines. *BMJ, 350:* h949.

Eaton, S (2016) Delivering person-centred care in long-term conditions. *Future Hospital Journal,* 3 (2): 128–31.

Economist Intelligence Unit (2015) *The 2015 Quality of Death Index.* Available online at: www.eiuperspectives.economist.com/healthcare/2015-quality-death-index

Edsberg, LE, Black, JM, Goldberg, M, McNichol, L, Moore, L and Sieggreen, M (2016) Revised National Pressure Ulcer Advisory Panel pressure injury staging system: revised pressure injury staging system. *Journal of Wound, Ostomy, and Continence Nursing, 43* (6): 585.

Egan, G (1998) *The Skilled Helper* (6th edn). Pacific Grove, CA: Brooks/Cole.

Egenes, KJ (2017) History of nursing. *Issues and Trends in Nursing: Essential Knowledge for Today and Tomorrow,* pp. 1–26. Sudbury, MA: Jones & Bartlett.

Elliott, A, Camacho, E, Campbell, F, Jankovic, D, Martyn St James, M, Kaltenthaler, E, Wong, R, Sculpher, M and Faria, R (2018) *Prevalence and Economic Burden of Medication*

Errors in the NHS in England. London: Policy Research Unit in Economic Methods of Evaluation in Health & Social Care Interventions (EEPRU).

Ellis, P (2016a) *Evidence-based Practice in Nursing* (3rd edn). London: Learning Matters/ SAGE.

Ellis, P (2016b) *Understanding Research for Nursing Students* (3rd edn). London: Learning Matters/SAGE.

Fallows, L, Matondo Mambu, J, Kemp, S, Campbell, B, Wansi, R, Adesina, A, Osei Owusu, A, Yusuf, O, Alewi, G, and Bello, A (2018) Creating a 'wish list' to prompt conversations on end-of-life care. *Nursing Times, 114* (1): 47–9.

Ferguson, C, DiGiacomo, M, Saliba, B. Green, J, Moorley, C, Wyllie, A and Jackson, D (2016) First year nursing students' experiences of social media during the transition to university: a focus group study. *Contemporary Nurse, 52* (5): 625–35.

Ferns, T and Chojnacka, I (2005) Nursing stereotypes: angels, swingers, matrons and sinners. *British Journal of Nursing, 14* (9): 1028.

Francis, R (2013) *Report of the Mid Staffordshire NHS Foundation Trust Public Inquiry.* London: The Stationery Office.

Fried, LP, Tangen, CM, Walston, J, Newman, AB, Hirsch, C, Gottdiener, J, Seeman, T, Tracy, R, Kop, WJ, Burke, G and McBurnie, MA (2001) Frailty in older adults: evidence for a phenotype. *The Journals of Gerontology Series A: Biological Sciences and Medical Sciences, 56* (3): M146–M157.

Fries, JF (2002) Aging, natural death, and the compression of morbidity. *Bulletin of the World Health Organization, 80* (3): 245–50.

Galloway, J (2011) Dignity, values, attitudes and person-centred care. In Hindle, A and Coates, A (eds) *Nursing Care of Older People.* Oxford: Oxford University Press, pp9–22.

Gibbs, G (1988) *Learning by Doing: A Guide to Learning and Teaching Methods.* Oxford: Oxford Brookes University, Further Education Unit.

Gillet, A (2018) *Using English for Academic Purposes for Students in Higher Education.* Available online at: www.uefap.net/ (accessed 8 February 2018).

Giminez, J (2007) *Writing for Nursing and Midwifery Students.* Basingstoke: Palgrave Macmillan.

Gimenez, J. (2008) Beyond the academic essay: discipline-specific writing in nursing and midwifery. *Journal of English for Academic Purposes, 7* (3) 151–64.

Gold Standards Framework (2009) Available online at: www.goldstandardsframework. org.uk/library

Gotts, JE and Matthay, MA (2016) Sepsis: pathophysiology and clinical management. *British Medical Journal, 353*: 1585.

Groenewegen, PP, Kerssens, JJ, Sixma, HJ, van der Eijk, I and Boerma, WG (2005) What is important in evaluating health care quality? An international comparison of user views. *BMC Health Services Research, 5* (1): 16.

Gross, A, Jones, RN, Habtemariam, DA, Fong, TG, Tommet, D, Quach, L, Schmitt, E, Yap, L and Inouye, SK (2012) Delirium and long-term cognitive trajectory among persons with dementia. *Archives of Internal Medicine, 172* (17): 1324–31.

Guerreiro, R, Escott-Price, V, Darwent, L, Parkkinen, L, Ansorge, O, Hernandez, DG et al. (2016) Genome-wide analysis of genetic correlation in dementia with Lewy bodies, Parkinson's and Alzheimer's diseases. *Neurobiology of Aging, 38* (Supplement C). DOI: 10.1016/j.neurobiolaging.2015.10.028.

Hafskjold, L, Sundler, AJ, Holstrom, IK, Sundling, V, van Dulmen, S and Eide, H (2015) A cross-sectional study on person-centred communication in the care of older people: the COMHOME study protocol. *BMJ Open, 5* (4), e007864.

Havighurst, RJ (1963) Successful aging. *Processes of Aging: Social and Psychological Perspectives, 1*: 299–320.

Hawthorn, M (2015) The importance of communication in sustaining hope at the end of life. *British Journal of Nursing, 24* (13): 702–5.

Health Foundation (2014) *Person-centred Care Made Simple.* London: The Health Foundation.

Higher Education Funding Council for England (HEFCE) (2017) *Open Access Research.* Available online at: https://webarchive.nationalarchives.gov.uk/20180103171825/http://www.hefce.ac.uk/rsrch/oa/Policy/

Hospice UK (2015) *Care after Death: Guidance for Staff Responsible for Care After Death.* Available online at: www.hospiceuk.org/what-we-offer/publications?cat=72e54312-4ccd-608d-ad24-ff0000fd3330

Howatson-Jones, L, Standing, M and Roberts, S (2015) *Patient Assessment and Care Planning in Nursing* (2nd edn). London: SAGE.

Huff, RM, Kline, MV and Peterson, DV (2014) *Health Promotion in Multicultural Populations: A Handbook for Practitioners and Students.* London: SAGE.

Hui, D, dos Santos, R, Chisholm, G, et al. (2014) Clinical signs of impending death in cancer patients, *Oncologist, 19* (6): 681–7.

Inouye, SK, Bogardus Jr, S, Charpentier, PA, Leo-Summers, L, Acampora, D, Holford, TR and Cooney Jr, LM (1999) A multicomponent intervention to prevent delirium in hospitalized older patients. *New England Journal of Medicine, 340* (9): 669–76.

International Council of Nurses (ICN) (2012) *Mission, Vision and Strategic Plan.* Geneva: ICN Mission.

Isaacs, B, (2002) *A Giant of Geriatric Medicine: Professor Bernard Isaacs (1924–1995).* British Geriatrics Society. Available online at: www.bgs.org.uk/geriatricmedicinearchive/bgsarchive/biographies/a-giant-of-geriatric-medicine-professor-bernard-isaacs-1924-1995 (accessed 26 July 2019).

Jakimowicz, S, Perry, L and Lewis, J (2017) An integrative review of supports, facilitators, and barriers to patient centred nursing in the intensive care unit. *Journal of Clinical Nursing, 26* (23–4): 4153–71.

Jarvis, C (2016) *Physical Examination & Health Assessment* (7th edn). St Louis, MO: Mosby/Elsevier.

Jayaweera, H (2014) *Health of Migrants in the UK: What Do We Know?* Available online at: www.migrationobservatory.ox.ac.uk/resources/briefings/health-of-migrants-in-the-uk-what-do-we-know/ (accessed 14 November 2017).

Johnson, M, Jefferies, D and Langdon, R (2010) The Nursing and Midwifery Content Audit Tool (NMCAT): a short nursing documentation audit tool. *Journal of Nursing Management, 18* (7): 832–45.

Kane, M and Cook, L (2013) *Dementia 2013: The Hidden Voice of Loneliness.* Alzheimer's Society. Available online at: www.alzheimers.org.uk/sites/default/files/migrate/downloads/dementia_2013_the_hidden_voice_of_loneliness.pdf

Kaukonen, KM, Bailey, M, Suzuki, S, Pilcher, D and Bellomo, R (2014) Mortality related to severe sepsis and septic shock among critically ill patients in Australia and New Zealand, 2000–2012. *JAMA, 311* (13): 1308–16.

Keeble, E, Roberts, H, Williams, C, Van Oppen, J and Conroy, S (2019) Poor outcomes of even brief hospital admissions among frail older people: a role for secondary prevention of frailty crises in the community? *British Journal of General Practice.*

Kelly, C (2008) Memory clinics. *Psychiatry, 7* (2): 61–3.

Keogh, B (2013) Review into the quality of care and treatment provided by 14 hospital trusts in England: overview report. London: NHS England.

King's Fund (2012) *Leadership and Engagement for Improvement in the NHS: Together We Can.* London: The King's Fund. Available online at: www.kingsfund.org.uk/sites/default/files/field/field_publication_file/leadership-for-engagement-improvement-nhs-final-review2012.pdf (accessed 2 May 2018).

King's Fund (2013) *Time to Think Differently.* London: The King's Fund. Available online at: www.kingsfund.org.uk/projects/time-think-differently (accessed 10 November 2017).

Kitwood, T (1997) On being a person. *Dementia Reconsidered: The Person Comes First,* pp. 7–19. Buckingham: Open University Press.

Leach, MJ (2008) Planning: a necessary step in clinical care. *Journal of Clinical Nursing 17* (13): 1728–34.

Leadership Alliance for the Care of Dying People (2014) 'One chance to get it right'. Available online at: https://assets.publishing.service.gov.uk/government/uploads/system/uploads/attachment_data/file/323188/One_chance_to_get_it_right.pdf

Levett-Jones, T, Hoffman, K, Dempsey, J, Jeong, SYS, Noble, D, Norton, CA, Roche, J and Hickey, N (2010) The 'five rights' of clinical reasoning: an educational model to enhance nursing students' ability to identify and manage clinically 'at risk' patients. *Nurse Education Today, 30* (6): 515–20.

Lillyman, S and Bruce, M (2016) Palliative care for people with dementia: a literature review. *International Journal of Palliative Nursing, 22* (2): 76–81. DOI: 10.12968/ijpn.2016.22.2.76.

Luft, J (1961) The Johari Window: a graphic model of awareness in interpersonal relations. *NTL Human Relations Training News, 5*: 6–7.

Maggie's (2018) *Why Maggie's programme of support works.* Available online from: www. maggiescentres.org (accessed 30 April 2018).

Maher, D and Hemming, L (2014) Understanding patient and family: holistic assessment in palliative care. *British Journal of Community Nursing, 10* (7).

Manley, K, Hills, V and Marriot, S (2011) Person-centred care: principle of nursing practice D. *Nursing Standard, 25* (31): 35–7.

Marieb, EN and Brito, S (2018) *Anatomy & Physiology Coloring Workbook: A Complete Study Guide.* London: Pearson Education.

McCabe, C and Timmins, F (2016) Embracing healthcare technology: what is the way forward for nurse education? *Nurse Education in Practice, 21*: 104–6.

McCance, T and McCormack, B (2017) The person-centred practice framework. In McCormack, B and McCance, T (eds) *Person-centred Practice in Nursing and Healthcare,* pp36–65. Oxford: Oxford University Press.

McCance, T, Gribben, B, McCormack, B and Laird, EA (2013) Promoting person-centred practice within acute care: the impact of culture and context on a facilitated practice development programme. *International Practice Development Journal, 3* (1): 1–14.

McConnell, D, McCance, T and Melby, V (2016) Exploring person-centredness in emergency departments: a literature review. *International Emergency Nursing, 26*: 38–46.

McCormack, B and McCance, TV (2006) Development of a framework for person-centred nursing. *Journal of Advanced Nursing, 56*: 472–9.

McCormack, B and McCance, T (2010) *Person-centred Nursing: Theory, Models and Methods.* Edinburgh: Queen Margaret University.

McEwen, M and Wills, EM (2018) *Theoretical Basis for Nursing.* New York: Lippincott Williams & Wilkins.

McKendry, S (2016) *Critical Thinking Skills for Healthcare.* Abingdon: Routledge.

McMahon, S, Home, NLC and Holywood, CD (2019) Pain assessment for people living with dementia in care homes. *Journal of the All Ireland Gerontological Nurses Association, 6* (1): 12–14.

McSherry, W (2006) *Making Sense of Spirituality in Nursing and Healthcare Practice: An Interactive Approach* (2nd edn). London: Jessica Kingsley.

Melin-Johansson, C, Palmqvist, R and Ronnberg, L (2017) Clinical intuition in the nursing process and decision-making—a mixed studies review. *Journal of Clinical Nursing, 26* (23–4): 3936–49.

Mid Staffordshire NHS Foundation Trust Public Inquiry (Great Britain) (2013) *Report of the Mid Staffordshire NHS Foundation Trust Public Inquiry.* London: The Stationery Office.

Milligan, S (2011) Addressing the spiritual care needs of people near the end of life. *Nursing Standard (through 2013), 26* (4): 47.

Minardi, H and Riley, M (1997) *Communication in Health Care: A Skills-based Approach.* London: Butterworth-Heinemann.

Moorley, C, Cahill, S and Corcoran, N (2016) Stroke among African-Caribbean women: lay beliefs of risks and causes. *Journal of Clinical Nursing, 25* (3–4): 403–11.

Moorley, CR and Chinn, T (2014) Nursing and Twitter: creating an online community using hashtags. *Collegian, 21* (2): 103–9.

Nair, M and Peate, I (2013) *Fundamentals of Anatomy and Physiology.* Chichester: Wiley-Blackwell.

NANDA International (2012) *NURSING DIAGNOSES. Definitions and Classification 2012–2014.* Chichester: Wiley-Blackwell/John Wiley & Sons.

National End of Life Care Programme (2014) *Dying Matters: Planning for Your Future.* University of Nottingham. Available online at: www.ncpc.org.uk/sites/default/files/planning_for_your_future_updated_sept_2014%20%281%29.pdf

National Institute for Health and Care Excellence (NICE) (2004) *Improving Supportive and Palliative Care for Adults with Cancer.* NICE Guidelines.

National Institute for Health and Care Excellence (NICE) (2006) *Dementia: Supporting People with Dementia and Their Carers in Health and Social Care.* Available online at: www.scie.org.uk/publications/misc/dementia/dementia-understanding.pdf?res=true (accessed 4 April 2018).

National Institute for Health and Care Excellence (NICE) (2007) *Acutely Ill Patients in Hospital: Recognition of and Response to Acute Illness in Adults in Hospital.* London: NICE Clinical Guideline no. 50.

National Institute for Health and Care Excellence (NICE) (2010) *Delirium: Diagnosis, Prevention and Management.* Clinical Guideline no. 103. Available online at: www.nice.org.uk/CG103.

National Institute of Clinical Excellence (NICE) (2012) *Patient Experience in Adult NHS Services: Improving the Experience of Care for People Using Adult NHS Services.* Available online at: www.nice.org.uk/guidance/cg138/resources/patient-experience-in-adult-nhs-services-improving-the-experience-of-care-for-people-using-adult-nhs-services-pdf-35109517087429 (accessed 16 August 2019).

National Institute for Health and Care Excellence (NICE) (2015a) *Falls in Older People.* Available online at: www.nice.org.uk/guidance/qs86/resources/falls-in-older-people-pdf-2098911933637 (accessed 27 March 2019).

National Institute for Health and Care Excellence (NICE) (2015b) *Care of Dying Adults in the Last Days of Life.* Available online at: www.nice.org.uk/guidance/ng31

National Institute for Health and Care Excellence (NICE) (2017) Dementia diagnosis and assessment. Available online at: https://pathways.nice.org.uk/pathways/dementia-disability-and-frailty-in-later-life-mid-life-approaches-to-delay-or-prevent-onset

National Institute of Health and Care Excellence (NICE) (2018) *Patient Experience in Adult NHS Services: Improving the Experience of Care for People Using Adult NHS Services.* Available online at: www.nice.org.uk/guidance/cg138 (accessed 4 April 2018).

National Palliative and End of Life Care Partnership (2015) *Ambitions for Palliative and End of Life Care: A National Framework for Local Action 2015–2020* (September). Available online at: www.endoflifecareambitions.org.uk

National Patient Safety Agency (2009) *Root Cause Analysis: Patient Safety.* Available online at: www.nrls.npsa.nhs.uk

National Patient Safety Agency (2009) *Safety in Doses: Improving the Use of Medicines in the NHS.* London: NPSA. Available online at: www.nrls.npsa.nhs.uk

National Pressure Ulcer Advisory Panel (2016) Available online at: https://cdn.ymaws.com/npuap.siteym.com/resource/resmgr/npuap_pressure_injury_stages.pdf (accessed July 2019).

National Voices and The National Council for Palliative Care (NCPC) and NHS England (2015) *Every Moment Counts: A Narrative for Person Centred Coordinated Care for People Near the End of Life.* London: National Voices. Available online at: www.ncpc.org.uk/news/every-moment-counts-new-vision-coordinated-care-people-near-end-life-calls-brave-conversations

NHS Chaplaincy Guidelines (2015) *Promoting Excellence in Pastoral, Spiritual and Religious Care.* Available online at: www.england.nhs.uk/wp-content/uploads/2015/03/nhs-chaplaincy-guidelines-2015.pdf

NHS Digital (2017) NHS Confederation. NHS statistics facts and figures. Available online at: www.nhsconfed.org/resources/key-statistics-on-the-nhs

NHS England (2012) *The 6Cs.* Available online at: www.england.nhs.uk/leadingchange/about/the-6cs/ (accessed 8 April 2018).

NHS England (2014) *Five Year Forward View.* Leeds: NHS England.

NHS Improvement (2018) *Pressure Ulcer Core Curriculum.* London: NHS Improvement.

Nicol, J and Nyatanga, B (2017) *Palliative and End of Life Care in Nursing.* London: Sage.

Northedge, A (2005) *The Good Study Guide* (2nd edn). Milton Keynes: The Open University Press.

Nouye, S, van Dyck, C, Alessi, C et al. (1990) Clarifying confusion: the confusion assessment method. *Annals of Internal Medicine, 113* (12): 941–8.

Nursing and Midwifery Council (NMC) (2010) *Standards for Pre-registration Nursing Education.* London: NMC.

Nursing and Midwifery Council (NMC) (2015) *The Code: Professional Standards of Practice and Behaviour for Nurses and Midwives.* London: NMC.

Nursing and Midwifery Council (NMC) (2018) *Future Nurse: Standards of Proficiency for Registered Nurses.* Available online at: www.nmc.org.uk/globalassets/sitedocuments/education-standards/print-friendly-future-nurse-proficiencies.pdf

Nursing and Midwifery Council (NMC) (2018) *The Code. Professional Standards of Practice and Behaviour for Nurses, Midwives and Nursing Associates.* London: NMC.

Nyatanga, B (2016) How do we achieve a good death? *British Journal of Community Nursing, 21* (10): 531.

O'Brien, M, Andrews, K and Spires, A (2011) *An Introduction to Medicines Management in Nursing.* Exeter: Learning Matters.

Office for National Statistics (2017) *Deaths Registered in England and Wales, 2016.* Available online at: www.ons.gov.uk/peoplepopulationandcommunity/birthsdeathsandmarriages/deaths/bulletins/deathsregistrationsummarytables/2016 (accessed December 2017).

Oh, ES, Fong, TG, Hshieh, TT and Inouye, SK (2017) Delirium in older persons: advances in diagnosis and treatment. *JAMA, 318* (12): 1161–74.

O'Mahony, D, O'Sullivan, D, Byrne, S, O'Connor, MN, Ryan, C and Gallagher, P (2015) STOPP/START criteria for potentially inappropriate prescribing in older people: version 2. *Age and Ageing, 44*(2): 213–18.

Orem, D (1980) *Nursing: Concepts of Practice.* New York: McGraw-Hill.

Orlando, IJ (1961) *The Dynamic Nurse–Patient Relationship: Function, Process, and Principles.* New York: Putnam.

Patel, JV, Vyas, A, Cruickshank, JK, Prabhakaran, D, Hughes, E and Reddy, KS (2006) Impact of migration on coronary heart disease risk factors: comparison of Gujaratis in Britain and their contemporaries in villages of origin in India. *Atherosclerosis, 185* (2): 297–306.

Payne, E and Whittaker, L (2006) *Developing Essential Study Skills* (2nd edn). Harlow: Pearson Education.

Pearce, E (1971) *A General Textbook of Nursing* (18th edn). London: Faber & Faber.

Peate, I (2016) *Fundamentals of Anatomy and Physiology: For Nursing and Healthcare Students.* Chichester: John Wiley & Sons.

Peplau, HE (1992) Interpersonal relations: a theoretical framework for application in nursing practice. *Nursing Science Quarterly, 5* (1): 13–18.

Pesut, B and Greig, M (2018) Resources for educating, training, and mentoring nurses and unregulated nursing care providers in palliative care: a review and expert consultation. *Journal of Palliative Medicine, 21* (S1): S–50.

Petro-Yura, H and Walsh, M (1967) *The Nursing Process.* Washington, DC: Catholic University of America Press.

Planetree (n.d.) *About Us.* Available online at: http://planetree.org/about-planetree/ (accessed 8 April 2018).

Porth, C (2011) *Essentials of Pathophysiology* (3rd edn). Philadelphia, PA; London: Wolters Kluwer/Lippincott Williams & Wilkins.

Prime Minister's Challenge on Dementia (2015) Available online at: www.gov.uk/government/publications/prime-ministers-challenge-on-dementia-2020/prime-ministers-challenge-on-dementia-2020 (accessed 15 November 2017).

Public Health England (2016) *Faith at End of Life: A Resource for Professionals, Providers and Commissioners Working in Communities.* Available online at: www.gov.uk/government/publications/faith-at-end-of-life-public-health-approach-resource-for-professionals

Public Health England (2017) *Trends in Morbidity and Behavioural Risk Factors: Morbidity by Age.* Available online at: www.gov.uk/government/publications/health-profile-for-england/chapter-3-trends-in-morbidity-and-behavioural-risk-factors (accessed 28 November 2017).

Public Health England (2018) *Falls: Applying All Our Health.* Available online at: www.gov.uk/government/publications/falls-applying-all-our-health/falls-applying-all-our-health (accessed 27.3.19)

Public Health England (2018) *Pressure Ulcers: Applying All Our Health.* Available online at: www.gov.uk/guidance/pressure-ulcers-applying-all-our-health (accessed 10 July 2019).

Rassin, RM (2010) Values grading among nursing students: differences between the ethnic groups. *Nurse Education Today, 30* (5): 458–63.

Rechel, B, Mladovsky, P, Ingleby, D, Mackenbach, JP and McKee, M (2013) Migration and health in an increasingly diverse Europe. *The Lancet, 381* (9873): 1235–45.

Robinson, L, Tang, E and Taylor, J (2015) Dementia: timely diagnosis and early intervention, *BMJ,* 350: h3029.

Rodda, J and Carter, J (2012) Cholinesterase inhibitors and memantine for symptomatic treatment of dementia. *BMJ, 344,* p.e2986.

Rogers, CR (1951) *Client-centred Therapy.* London: Constable.

Roper, N (1976) A model for nursing and nursology. *Journal of Advanced Nursing* (online), *1* (3), 219–27.

Roper, N, Logan, WW and Tierney, AJ (2000) *The Roper–Logan–Tierney Model of Nursing: Based on Activities of Living.* London: Elsevier Health Sciences.

Ross H, Tod, AM and Clarke, A (2015) Understanding and achieving person-centred care: the nurse perspective. *Journal of Clinical Nursing, 24* (9–10): 1223–33.

Rowe, JW and Kahn, RL (1997) Successful Aging. *The Gerontologist, 37* (4): 433–40.

Royal College of Nursing (RCN) (2009) *Royal College of Nursing Submission to the Prime Minister's Commission on Nursing and Midwifery.* London: RCN.

Royal College of Nursing (RCN) (2010) *Principles of Nursing Practice.* Available online at: www.rcn.org.uk/professional-development/principles-of-nursing-practice

Royal College of Nursing (RCN) (2014) *Defining Nursing.* Available online at: http://anaesthesiaconference.kiev.ua/downloads/definingnursing_2003.pdf

Royal College of Nursing (2015) *Accountability.* Available online at: https://rcni.com/hosted-content/rcn/first-steps/accountability

Royal College of Nursing (RCN) (2015) *Getting it Right Every Time: Fundamentals of Nursing Care at the End of Life.* Available online at: http://rcnendoflife.org.uk/communication/

Royal College of Physicians (RCP) (2017) *National Early Warning Score (NEWS) 2: Standardising the Assessment of Acute-illness Severity in the NHS.* Updated report of a working party. London: RCP.

Royal College of Psychiatrists (RCPsych) (2017) *National Audit of Dementia Care.* London: RCPsych.

Rubio-Valera, M, Pons-Vigues, M, Martinez-Andres, M, Moreno-Peral, P, Bereguera, A and Fernandex, A (2014) Barriers and facilitators for the implementation of primary prevention and health promotion activities in primary care: a synthesis through meta-ethnography. *PloS One*, 28 February.

Saba, VK and Taylor, SL (2007) Moving past theory: use of a standardized, coded nursing terminology to enhance nursing visibility. *Computers, Informatics, Nursing*, 25 (6): 324–31.

Salluh, JI, Wang, H, Schneider, EB, Nagaraja, N, Yenokyan, G, Damluji, A, Serafim, RB and Stevens, RD (2015) Outcome of delirium in critically ill patients: systematic review and meta-analysis. *BMJ*, *350*, p.h2538.

Schenker, Y, Fernandez, A, Sudore, R and Schillinger, D (2011) Interventions to improve patient comprehension in informed consent for medical and surgical procedures: a systematic review. *Medical Decision Making*, *31* (1): 151–73.

Shipley, SD (2010) Listening: a concept analysis. In *Nursing Forum*, 45 (2): 125–34. Malden, MA: Blackwell Publishing.

Silverman, J, Kurtz, S and Draper, J (2016) *Skills for Communicating with Patients*. Boca Raton, FL: CRC Press.

Singer, M, Deutschman, CS, Seymour, CW, Shankar-Hari, M, Annane, D, Bauer, M, Bellomo, R, Bernard, GR, Chiche, JD, Coopersmith, CM and Hotchkiss, RS (2016) The third international consensus definitions for sepsis and septic shock (sepsis-3). *JAMA*, *315* (8): 801–10.

Talbot, L and Verrinder, G (2009) *Promoting Health: The Primary Health Care Approach*. (4th edn). London: Elsevier.

Tavers, A and Taylor, V (2016) What are the barriers to initiating end-of-life conversations with patients in the last year of life? *International Journal of Palliative Nursing*, *22* (9): 454–62.

Taylor, P, Dowding, D and Johnson, M (2017) Clinical decision making in the recognition of dying: a qualitative interview study. *BMC Palliative Care*, *16* (11): 1–14.

Thackeray, R and Neiger, BL (2009) A multidirectional communication model: implications for social marketing practice. *Health Promotion Practice*, *10* (2): 171–5.

Thim, T, Krarup, NHV, Grove, EL, Rohde, CV and Løfgren, B (2012) Initial assessment and treatment with the Airway, Breathing, Circulation, Disability, Exposure (ABCDE) approach. *International Journal of General Medicine*, *5*: 117.

Todd, O, and Teale, E (2017) Delirium: a guide for the general physician. *Clinical Medicine*, *17* (1): 48. Available online at: https://search.proquest.com/docview/1865733736

Tuinman, A, de Greef, MH, Krijnen, WP, Paans, W and Roodbol, PF (2017) Accuracy of documentation in the nursing care plan in long-term institutional care. *Geriatric Nursing*, *38* (6): 578–83.

United Kingdom Central Council (UKCC) (1994) *The Future of Professional Practice: The Council's Standards for Education and Practice Following Registration*. London: UKCC.

Waller, S and Masterson, A (2015) Designing dementia-friendly hospital environments. *Future Hospital Journal*, 2 (1): 63–8.

Warren, J, Rohrer, J and Rossor, M (2013) Frontotemporal dementia. *BMJ*, 347. DOI: 10.1136/bmj.f4827.

Watson, J (1999) *Nursing: Human Science and Human Care: A Theory of Nursing.* Sudbury, MA: Jones & Bartlett.

Whitehead, D (2002) The academic writing experiences of a group of student nurses: a phenomenological study. *Journal of Advance Nursing, 38* (5): 498–506.

Wilson, B, Woollands, A and Barrett, D (2018) *Care Planning: A Guide for Nurses* (3rd edn). London: Routledge.

Wingate, U (2011) 'Argument!' helping students understand what essay writing is about. Elsevier.

Wise, J (2017) Vascular risk factors show link to development of Alzheimer's. *BMJ* (online), 357. DOI: 10.1136/bmj.j1847.

Wittenberg, E, Ferrell, BR, Goldsmith, J, Smith, T, Ragan, SL, Glajchen, MN and Handozo, G (2016) *Textbook of Palliative Care Communication.* Oxford: Oxford University Press.

World Health Organization (WHO) (1986) *The Ottawa Charter for Health Promotion: First International Conference on Health Promotion.* Ottawa, 21 November. Geneva: WHO.

World Health Organization (WHO) (2002) *Active Ageing: A Policy Framework.* Geneva: WHO.

Yildirim, MB and Ozkahraman, S (2011) Critical thinking in nursing process and education. *International Journal of Humanities and Social Science, 1* (13): 257–62.

Yura, H, Walsh, MB and Catholic University of America, School of Nursing (1973) *The Nursing Process: Assessing, Planning, Implementing, Evaluating.* New York: Appleton-Century-Crofts.

Zarb, P, Coignard, B, Griskeviciene, J, Muller, A, Vankerckhoven, V and Weist, K (2012) The European Centre for Disease Prevention and Control (ECDC) pilot point prevalence survey of healthcare-associated infections and antimicrobial use. *Eurosurveilance, 17* (46): 20316.

Index

Added to a page number 't' denotes a table and 'f' denotes a figure.

arterial vasoconstriction 127
arteries 116, 117f, 120–1, 126, 127
arterioles 126, 127
arthritis 236
article processing charges (APCs) 35
aspirin 178, 180, 188, 202
asplenia 75
assessment
  of patient urine 129
  of suitability of health resources 64
  see also patient assessment; risk assessment
assignments *see* essay writing
assumption of (mental) capacity 213
asthma 173, 187, 201
astrocytes 133
Atchley, R. 236
atrioventricular bundle (bundle of His) 122
atrioventricular node 122
attentive listening 220
attorneys 77, 246–7
audio-visual materials 44
Augmentin® 190
Australian Department of Social Services 152
autoimmune disease 75
autonomy (patient) 77, 147, 148, 152, 165, 223, 245

Baldwin, M.A. 210
Barry (case study) 20
β₂ receptors 187
behaviour 21
behavioural and psychological symptoms of dementia
  (BPSD) 243
being in place 156
being in relation 155
being with self 155
being in a social world 156
beliefs 25, 58, 78, 149, 152, 155
  see also religion
best interests (patient's) 18, 77, 84, 222
Best practice for providing excellent spiritual care (NHS,
  2015) 220
beta blockers 173, 201
Beth (case study) 144
bicarbonate (HCO₃) 126, 127, 128
bicarbonate ions 118
bile 137, 138
bioavailability 185, 189
biotransformation 181
Blackfriars Consensus (2014) 240
bladder (urinary) 125, 126, 127
blood brain barrier (BBB) 180–1, 187
blood buffers 118
blood filtration 125, 126–7
blood flow 121, 122, 178, 183, 202
blood osmolarity 128
blood pH 118, 128
blood pressure 83, 88, 104, 121, 128
Boards for Nursing 14
bolus 137
books (monographs) 35, 42
  see also e-books and journals

boundaries, professional 21, 22, 25, 30, 68
Bowman's capsule 125
brainstem 130–1
brainstorming 46–7
brand names (drug) 190
British Association Parenteral and Enteral Nutrition
  (BAPEN) 98–9
British Heart Foundation 63
British National Formulary 174, 190
British Nurses Association 13
bronchioles 116, 117
bronchoconstriction 201
bronchodilation 187
Brooke, J. 59, 153
Bruce, M. 246
building design, and patient experience 156, 245
bundle of His 122
Burns, A. 239

caecum 135, 138
Calgary–Cambridge model 211–12
Calvin (case study) 92–3, 99, 106–7, 110
cancer 236
capability (patient) 148
capillaries 117f, 120–1, 125, 126, 127
carbamazepine 202
carbon dioxide (CO₂) 117, 118, 128
carbonic acid (H₂CO₃) 118, 128
cardiac arrest 134
cardiac failure 183, 188, 202, 236
cardiovascular system 120–1, 127
care
  after death 225–7
  and communication *see* communication
  as a core value 18
  cultural insensitivity 235
  documentation 84–5
  environment 150, 153, 154, 156, 249
  evaluation 25, 83, 84, 89, 166–7
  gender-matched 166
  models 24–8
  of older people 238
  patient's right to ask questions about 84
  process *see* nursing, process(es)
  quality of 9, 10, 84, 156
  reflection on 83–4
  see also intermediate care; palliative and end-of-life
    care; patient-centred care; person-centred care
care coordinators 242
care plans 150–1
  dementia 242
  fall prevention 110–11
  ownership 161
  person-centred 157
  standards 161
  writing 160–3
Care Quality Commission (CQC) 161, 215
career pathway 14
carrier/transport mechanisms (drug) 189
catalogues (library) 38
central nervous system (CNS) 130–1, 132f, 133